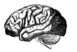

ANDERS HANSEN

THE *REAL*

HAPPY PILL

POWER UP YOUR BRAIN BY MOVING YOUR BODY

TRANSLATION BY GUN PENHOAT

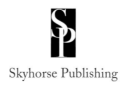

Skyhorse Publishing

Skyhorse Publishing books may be purchased in bulk at special discounts for sales promotion, corporate gifts, fund-raising, or educational purposes. Special editions can also be created to specifications. For details, contact the Special Sales Department, Skyhorse Publishing, 307 West 36th Street, 11th Floor, New York, NY 10018 or info@skyhorsepublishing.com.

Skyhorse® and Skyhorse Publishing® are registered trademarks of Skyhorse Publishing, Inc.®, a Delaware corporation.

Visit our website at www.skyhorsepublishing.com.

10 9 8 7 6 5 4 3 2 1

Library of Congress Cataloging-in-Publication Data is available on file.

Cover design by Lisa Zachrisson
Cover photo credit: Lisa Zachrisson
Illustrations by Lisa Zachrisson

Print ISBN: 978-1-5107-2298-9
Ebook ISBN: 978-1-5107-2299-6

Printed in China

For all its material advantages,
the sedentary life has left us edgy,
unfulfilled. CARL SAGAN

Dedicated to:
Hans-Åke Hansen (1940–2011)
Vanja Hansen & Björn Hansen

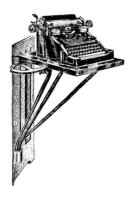

CONTENTS

FOREWORD—EXERCISE YOUR BRAIN

Make two fists and join them together side by side. This is the size of your brain. It weighs about the same as a carton of milk. Imagine something this small containing everything you have ever felt and experienced. All your personality traits. Everything you have ever learned. All your memories—from your first, faint mental images of a summer vacation when you were three; through your childhood and teenage years; to your current, grownup life where you are now reading these very words.

Everything is stored in that lump, which is the universe's most complex structure that we know of and which consumes no more energy than a light bulb. Whoever isn't fascinated by the brain can't be intrigued by much more.

While we've known for some time now how the body's other organs work, the brain has remained a mystery—up until now. Thanks to recently developed research tools, our knowledge has made great leaps these past decades. We have begun to understand, in detail, how the brain functions; today, few call into question that we don't merely have a brain, but that in fact we *are* our brain.

However, just because brain research has given us a biological glimpse at human characteristics doesn't mean that your fate is sealed and unchangeable. Studies have brought to light just how fantastically malleable the brain can be, not only in children but also in adults. New brain cells develop constantly. Connections are created, and connections disappear. Everything you do, down to every thought you have, modifies the brain a little bit. Your brain is more akin to modeling clay than china.

So how do you shape this "modeling clay"? Well, there are few things as important for your brain as moving your body. Not only do you feel better when you're physically active; your concentration, memory, creativity, and resistance to stress are also affected. You're able to process information more quickly—so you *think* faster—and become more adept at mobilizing intellectual resources as needed. You have access to an extra "mental gear" to help you focus when things get hectic around you and to stay calm when your thoughts start racing. In fact, physical activity even seems to increase your level of intelligence.

Doesn't that sound strange? After all, if we want stronger arms, we train our arms, not our legs. The same should to apply to the brain: if we want a brain that functions better, surely we ought to train with crosswords, memory exercises, and other brain gymnastics? As it turns out, that's not true. Research clearly indicates that memory exercises, Sudoku, and crosswords don't come close to boosting the brain in the same positive way as does engaging in regular physical activity. Surprisingly, the brain seems to be the organ that benefits the most from our being in motion.

In this book, I'm going to show you the huge impact exercise and training have on your brain—and explain the reasons why. Some of the results are noticeable immediately—as in, right after you've been for a walk or a run—while others require regular training for at least one year to take effect. I will also describe what you need to do specifically to achieve the outcomes and mental advantages that research has shown physical activity provides—benefits that amount to no less than a mental upgrade. Enjoy!

Anders Hansen

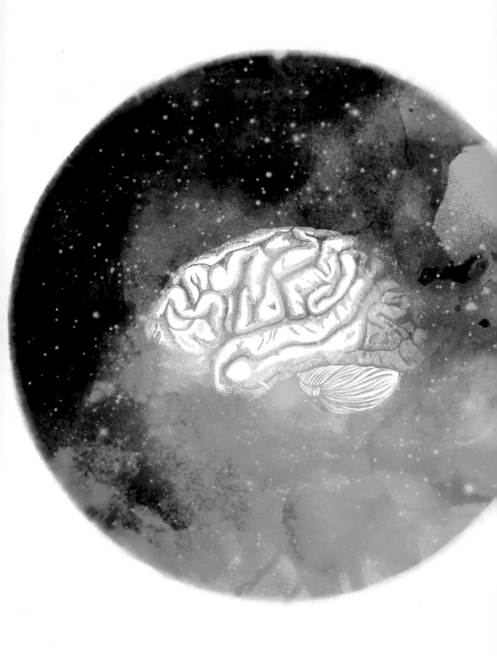

1. YOUR CHANGEABLE BRAIN

*The chief function of the body
is to carry the brain around*
THOMAS A. EDISON

I magine that you're sitting in a time machine and you've cranked the year back to 10,000 BC. The machine starts clanging, and suddenly you're hurtled thousands of years back in time. You nervously step out of the capsule and look around you. A group of people dressed in animal hides are standing there, and they seem surprised to see you.

What is your first impression of them? That they're primitive "cave dwellers" who, at best, might be able to hunt down an animal and kill it but are otherwise unable to show any hint of advanced thought? It might be easy to reach this conclusion, but in fact you and they are very much alike. Of course, they don't speak the same language, and they have a completely different set of experiences, but overall they function quite similarly to you. They possess the same cognitive abilities and feelings you do. We humans have not changed all that much, really, over the past twelve thousand years.

By contrast, your lifestyle has undergone immense transformation in only one hundred years, and if you look back twelve thousand years, the degree of change is unbelievable. You live in material comfort and make use of technical tools the likes of which your ancient predecessors could not conceive of in their wildest dreams. You exist in entirely different social environments. You probably meet as many fresh faces in a single week as they would over the course of their entire lifetime.

There is also another fundamental difference between your way of life and that of your ancestors: they move considerably more than you do. Taken in historical context, they are not alone in doing this. Over millions of years, our ancestors were significantly more physically active than we are today, and the reason is simple: throughout most of human history, it has been necessary to be physically active to procure food and to survive. Consequently, not only is our body built for movement, so is our brain.

One hundred years might seem like an eternity—let alone twelve thousand years—but from a biological perspective, it's no longer than the blink of an eye. Evolution often requires considerably more time before big changes appear in any species, and this applies to us humans, too. Our brain hasn't changed significantly, whether in one century or over twelve thousand years. Despite the enormous transformations we have made to our lifestyle that have removed us further and further from the life we were designed for, our brains are still living in the savanna— where our hunter-gatherer ancestors lived many years ago. That is true especially when it comes down to how much we move. Even though we don't need to hunt for our food and can now order our groceries online, our brain still runs more efficiently if we live a little more like our ancestors did—when we move our bodies.

EXERCISE AND TRAINING PRODUCES A MORE EFFICIENT BRAIN

I've read thousands of studies over the years, and if I had to pick one that fascinated me the most, one that not only changed my view of medicine and health but also, to a certain degree, my view of life in general, it would be the study in which the brains of about one hundred sixty-year-old human test subjects were examined by MRI.

MRI—Magnetic Resonance Imaging—is nothing short of a technical miracle for brain researchers; it is a tool that has truly opened us up to another world. Today, thanks to MRI, we can "lift the lid" and look inside the cranium to get a picture, in real time, of how the brain works while we think and perform different tasks, at no risk of injury to the person being examined.

The goal of this one specific study was to understand the effects of aging on the brain, because our brain, just like our skin, heart, and lungs, gets old. But *how* does it age, really? And are we doomed to go through the aging process with no means of influencing its course, or are we able to alter it in any way, perhaps by engaging in regular physical activity? This is what researchers began to suspect after animal trials demonstrated that brains of caged mice that ran on a wheel, compared to those that didn't, tended to age slower.

For the study's authors to answer these questions, the sixty-year-old participants were split into two groups: in the first, the subjects took regular walks a few times a week over the course of one year; and in the second, the people met as often as the other group but performed easy exercises that did not elevate their heart rate.

The test subjects' brains were examined by MRI prior to the onset of the study, as well as one year after the study, whether they were in the group that took the walks or did the easy exercises.

To track the participants' brain processes, these MRIs took place while the subjects were performing a concurrent set of psychological tests. The scans revealed how different parts of the brain were being activated and exposed how areas in the temporal lobe worked together with areas in the occipital lobe and the frontal lobe, in what appeared to be a sophisticated network.

However, the most telling revelation lay not in the results per se, but in the contrast those results showed between the study's two test groups.

The participants who walked didn't just get in better shape over the course of the year; they also developed a more effective brain. The MRIs showed that the connections between the lobes had strengthened, most notably between the temporal lobe to both frontal and occipital lobes. In short, different sections of the brain were better integrated with one another, which in turn meant, quite simply, that the entire organ functioned more efficiently.

Somehow the physical activity (i.e., the walks) had had a positive impact on the brain's connectivity pattern.

When the data from the sixty-year-olds' tests were compared to that of tests performed on younger subjects, it was impossible to reach any other conclusion: the brains of participants who had been physically active appeared younger. They did not look as though they had aged during the year; instead, they seemed to have become biologically stronger, the most striking effect being the connection between the frontal and the temporal lobe, which is in fact the area of the brain that tends to be most affected by aging. Seeing improvement in that area indicated that the aging process had stalled.

In addition to yielding measurable results, more importantly those regular walks made a real, practical difference. Psychological tests showed that the set of cognitive functions called *executive control* or *executive function*, which among other things include the abilities to take initiative, plan, and have attentional control, showed improvement in the group of test subjects who walked.

Simply put, this discovery means that the brain works more efficiently in people who are physically active, and that the detrimental effects of aging can be halted or even reversed to make the brain more energetic.

Take a minute to think about what you've just read. Go over it again. If that isn't enough motivation to start moving, I don't know what is. You know that you'll improve your stamina by running and that you'll develop bigger muscles by lifting weights, but you probably weren't aware that exercise and training can also bring about changes in your brain—changes that are not only measurable by modern medical technology, but are also extremely important to optimal cognitive function.

We're going to examine these changes in more detail later in this book. But first we're going to look at how the brain works, and then we'll see how it can be made to operate better.

YOUR INNER UNIVERSE

The brain has shown itself to be more malleable than we have previously thought. What you have inside your cranium isn't some type of advanced computer with genetically preprogrammed functions, destined to develop in a certain way. The brain is far more complex than that. It contains approximately one hundred billion (100,000,000,000) brain cells. Each cell can connect to tens of thousands of other cells, which means that the number of possible connections in the brain totals at least one hundred thousand billion. That is one thousand (1,000) times more than the number of stars in the milky way or galaxies in the universe. To say that you have your own universe inside your skull might sound somewhat New Age-y, but the inner universe is what this is all about.

Old brain cells die, and new cells are created continuously. Connections are made between the cells and become disconnected if not in use. The strength of those connections changes in time depending on how the brain redesigns its architecture. You can look at the brain as a highly sophisticated ecosystem in a state of constant flux. It keeps changing throughout life, and not only when you are a child or when you learn something new. Each sensation you experience, every thought you have—everything leaves a trace and changes you a little. The brain you have today is not quite the same as the one you had yesterday. The brain is a continuous *work in progress.*

It is not the number of brain cells or connections that is key

Some believe that the amount of brain cells or the size of the brain determines whether a brain functions well. That is not correct. The most telling example is Albert Einstein, whose brain was neither bigger nor heavier than the average brain. Einstein's brain weighed 1,230 grams (2.7 pounds), compared to 1,350 grams (2.97 pounds) of the average man's brain and to the average woman's, which weighs approximately 100 grams (3.5 ounces) less.

For a long time, I believed that it was the number of connections between brain cells that determined the brain's capacity, but that's

> *Every impression and every thought leaves a trace, and changes your brain a little bit.*

not right, either. Two-year-old children have significantly more connections between brain cells than adults have. As a child grows, the amount of connections decrease. This process is called *pruning*, and it's estimated that up to twenty billion (20,000,000,000) connections disappear *every 24 hours* from the age of two up to adolescence. The brain weeds out unused connections to make room for the ones that carry a signal. This can be summarized as: *Neurons that fire together wire together.*

But if neither the number of brain cells nor the amount of connections between them determines the quality of a brain, what does? The answer is that when we stay busy doing different things—biking, reading a book, or planning what to have for dinner, for instance—the brain uses a type of program that is called a *functional network*. You have a program for swimming, another one for biking, and a third for writing your signature. Everything you do is dependent on these networks, which are all basically built by a collection of brain cells that are connected to one another. A program can integrate cells from many different areas of the brain. And for it to run optimally—to enable you to swim, ride a bike, or sign something—it is necessary for the brain's different areas to be closely interconnected.

Practice makes perfect—and it makes more agile brain programs

For example, imagine that you'd like to learn to play a simple tune on the piano. Many different areas in the brain must work together to make that possible. For a start, you'll need to see the piano keys. A signal goes from the eyes through the optic nerve to the primary visual cortex in the occipital lobe. Simultaneously, the brain motor cortex must coordinate the movements of your hands and fingers. The auditory cortex processes sound information and sends it on to areas called the *association areas*, in the temporal and parietal lobes. The information eventually reaches the frontal lobe, the seat of your consciousness and higher brain functions, and you become aware of what you are playing and can correct any wrong notes you play. All this hub of activity, just to play a simple piano tune!

All these areas in the visual and auditory centrums, the motor cortex, and the parietal and frontal lobes are part of the brain's program for playing music. The more you practice, the better you become at it, and the more efficiently the program runs in your brain. At the beginning, it will take a great deal of effort to play the tune. The program is inefficient and awkward and requires that big chunks of the brain be fully engaged in the task. That's why you'll experience playing the piano as mentally taxing, and you will need to focus hard to accomplish the task.

In time, as you continue practicing, it will become easier. Once you've put in a tremendous amount of work, you will be able to play the tune while thinking of something different. The brain's program for playing the tune has now become efficient at transferring information: a repeated signal through the network has strengthened the connection— *neurons that fire together wire together*. In the end, less and less mental effort will be required, and you'll be able to play the tune without giving it a second thought.

As the program for playing the tune activates cells from different areas of the brain, those different areas need to be closely connected for the program to run well. We can compare it to a computer, where all the different components need to be connected in order to work. If the connections are bad, the computer won't run, even if each input works well independently.

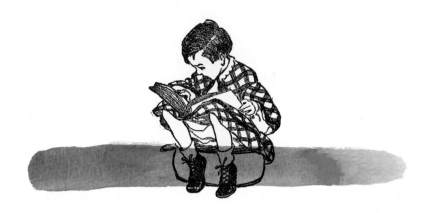

AS KIDS, WE'RE ALL LINGUISTIC GENIUSES

The fact that connections between brain cells disappear when we are children has lifelong consequences. A child born in Sweden has all the prerequisites for learning to speak fluently in Japanese without any trace of an accent—provided the child is reared in an environment in which Japanese is spoken. On the other hand, learning to speak fluent Japanese without an accent as an adult is next to impossible for most of us. No matter how much we practice, a native-born Japanese will always be able to detect an accent in our speech.

Spoken language features certain sounds that we have enormous difficulty replicating once we're adults, and that's because our prerequisites are missing. The brain connections that handle those sounds begin to disappear during childhood because we never hear those sounds being articulated. Once the connections are gone, we have closed the door to those abilities, neurologically speaking, for the rest of our lives. While we're kids, however, we are all little linguistic geniuses.

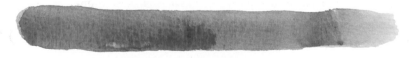

So it's not the brain with lots of brain cells or many connections between cells that functions best, but rather the one in which the different areas—the frontal lobe and the parietal lobe, for example—are closely interconnected, thus possessing everything that's required to run effective programs. As you've already read in the beginning of this chapter, physical activity can create stronger connections between the different parts of the brain. This connectivity is the basis for a number of positive effects your brain experiences when you move your body, many of which you will read about in this book.

The connections reveal how you live your life

It may sound a bit strange that different areas of the brain can all be, to different degrees, well connected to one another, but research has shown that this could in fact be an important reason why cognitive abilities vary among people. Fascinating findings have recently been uncovered in this specific area of research.

For example, advanced brain testing on hundreds of individuals has revealed that different parts of the brain are closely interconnected in the people with sets of qualities deemed positive, such as good memory function and power of concentration, higher education, and carefulness with alcohol and tobacco. In subjects with "negative" qualities, such as poor anger management and the tendency to abuse alcohol and drugs, an opposite pattern has been observed: these areas of the brain are badly linked to one another.

That many positive qualities leave an identical imprint on the brain, and that negative qualities seem to make the opposite type of mark, implies that there is a "positive-negative axis" along which we could all be placed, depending on how we live. Scientists who have performed this study believe that you can see how a person leads his or her life, roughly, by looking at his or her brain's connectivity pattern. And is there anything else that's considered a positive sign

It looks like it actually may be possible to see, roughly, what kind of life a person leads by looking at his or her brain's connections.

along that positive-negative axis apart from good memory, higher education, and caution with addictive substances? Indeed, there is. It's being in good physical shape.

Judgmental research?

You might believe that this type of research is judgmental or elitist; after all, the mere fact that we are talking about a "positive-negative axis" suggests a sort of ranking of people. I completely understand how it could be interpreted that way, but I also believe that such an interpretation misses the point. Our inherent qualities are not what primarily affects our brain's connectivity pattern, nor where we are situated along the positive-negative axis. Instead, it is our lifestyle. Through the choices we make, we can change our brain's operating mode on a more fundamental level than previously thought. It isn't only our brain that decides how we think and act; our thoughts and actions can also modify our brain and how it works. It is we who run our brain, not the other way around. From this perspective, it is clear that perhaps the most important thing to improve the connection between the different parts of our brain is regular physical exercise; being in good physical condition produces a positive reading on the positive-negative axis.

THE BRAIN CHANGES THROUGHOUT LIFE—NEUROPLASTICITY

"I wish I had learned to play an instrument as a kid; now it's too late." Many of us might have had this thought at one time or another. The truth is the brain is extremely malleable during childhood, making learning everything, from languages to motor skills, swift and natural. But why is it that a child's brain can learn so much in such a short time, with little obvious effort?

A young child must quickly learn to navigate in the world. In the brain, this is evident from the cells' enormous ability to not only create connections with one another, but also to break them off (i.e., *pruning*). This happens at a rate of speed that, as you've noticed, will never come back later in life. However, the brain's capacity for change, which in scientific parlance is referred to as *neuroplasticity*, is perhaps its most important quality, because even if its flexibility is never as great as when we were children, it doesn't vanish entirely. It's still there—even in adults, even in eighty-year-olds. To see exactly how influenceable and changeable the brain is in an adult, we're going to look at what happened to Michelle Mack, a forty-two-year-old American woman whose remarkable life story has changed our understanding of what the human brain is truly capable of.

The woman who only had half her brain

Michelle Mack was born in Virginia in November 1973. As early as a few weeks after her birth, her parents noticed that something was not right. Michelle was unable to steady her gaze and couldn't move her limbs normally, especially her right arm and leg. Her parents brought her to numerous specialists to examine her eyes and to see if she had cerebral palsy, which was not the case. None of the neurologists they consulted could explain Michelle's symptoms, and neither could an X-ray of her brain. In the early 1970s, our modern technologies (i.e., the CAT scan [Computerized Axial Tomography] and MRI [Magnetic Resonance Imaging]) were still in the early developmental stages. At the age of three, Michelle still wasn't walking, and she could hardly speak. At this point, her physician recommended that another X-ray be scheduled since medical diagnostic techniques had advanced since her first examination. The result of the

YOUR LIFESTYLE SHAPES YOUR BRAIN

The debate on whether our genes or our environment shapes us has ebbed and flowed over time, often from one extreme point of view to another more stringent opinion. Today we know that it is, of course, *neither* our genetic makeup *nor* our environment that decides our fate exclusively, but a combination of both. We also know that genes and environment are closely interwoven, whereby environment affects our genes—our DNA (Deoxyribonucleic Acid)—through biological mechanisms that are incredibly complex.

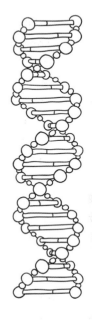

A few numbers clearly illustrate that it isn't only your genetic makeup that decides on its own how your brain will develop and how you will turn out as a human being. You possess approximately 23,000 genes. You also have about 100 billion brain cells that, in turn, have around 100,000 billion connections between them. Your 23,000 genes can't possibly hold sway over those 100,000 billion connections. Quite simply, the brain is far too complex to be governed by an exact predetermined genetic program that is in charge of the brain's development throughout life.

Your genes set the stage for how your brain cells are created and die, and how they connect and disconnect from one another. Exactly how this happens, which characteristics you develop, and how you function mentally will be influenced by your life experiences—by what type of environment you live in and not least by what lifestyle you adopt.

The aspect of our lifestyle that this book is all about—physical exercise—is, naturally, not the only factor in how our brain develops. However, research shows that it plays a pivotal role and is way more important than most of us can fathom.

CAT scan performed in 1977 shocked Michelle's parents, as well as her physicians. Michelle Mack was missing the entire left side of her brain. She was living with only half a brain, probably due to something that had happened to her while she was still an embryo.

One possibility is that Michelle had suffered a stroke before birth; another is that her left carotid artery had been blocked, depriving the left side of the brain of blood. No one could provide a definitive answer, but one thing was crystal clear: more than 90 percent of the left side of Michelle's brain was missing.

The left side of the brain is commonly referred to as the analytical and rational part of the brain—the seat of mathematical and linguistic thinking—while the right side is the artistic and creative part. Even though we now realize that this divvying up is an oversimplification of things, it isn't too far from reality. Bearing in mind the set of responsibilities held by the left side of the brain, many of Michelle's difficulties suddenly made sense. Her inability to speak properly could be explained by the missing linguistic part of her brain. And since the left side of the brain is also in charge of the mobility of the right side of the body (and vice versa), it's no wonder she had trouble moving her right arm and leg.

However, it isn't Michelle Mack's first years of life that are fascinating, but rather what happened to her later. She successively developed the abilities she had been lacking, at a rate that her physicians had not dared hope for. She learned to walk, speak, and read and otherwise developed somewhat normally, if a little more slowly, than most of her peers.

Today, Michelle lives a normal life in many ways and works part-time in her parish. Her ability to find words is mostly normal, even though that function is typically found in the part of the brain that's missing for Michelle. Although mobility in right arm and leg is still limited, she has no problem walking.

Tests have shown that Michelle has some difficulty with abstract thinking, but she is endowed with a phenomenal memory for detail.

This comes with a highly unusual skill: she can immediately answer what weekday corresponds to a randomly selected date. For instance, if Michelle is asked what day of the week the 18th of March, 2010, falls on, she'll answer "Thursday" almost instantly.

The right half of Michelle's brain has taken over the handling of many tasks that her left brain would normally be dealing with. We know from past studies that this could be done on a smaller scale, but few had speculated that such a massive restructuring of the brain, one that could compensate for a missing half, was possible. The rewiring of Michelle's brain is so extensive that it actually looks a bit crowded in her brain's right half. In fact, Michelle has issues with visuospatial orientation (i.e., the ability to judge distance and spatial orientation). Visuospatial orientation is normally found in the right part of the brain (which is intact in Michelle), but it is believed that since her brain's right side is pulling double duty—handling responsibilities for the right and the missing left side—there just isn't enough room in there.

It's also probably no accident that Michelle can immediately match a specific date to its corresponding day of the week. The two halves of our brain work as a kind of "Jante's Shield" (i.e., a preserver of uniformity) on each other. One side of the brain can't simply compensate for what the other half lacks; it must also restrain the other half if it grows too strong within a certain area so that we achieve balance in our cerebral abilities. This means that most of us acquire reasonable abilities in many areas instead of becoming extremely adept at some, and very poor at others. If the halves of the brain are unable to communicate, the equilibrium might be lost and certain abilities may blossom, often to the detriment of others.

A human Google

This is exactly what is believed to have happened to Kim Peek, an American man and the inspiration for Dustin Hoffman's role as Raymond Babbitt in the movie *Rain Man*. Peek was born with an injury to the *corpus callosum*, a band of nerve fibers. This band is the part of the brain that forms the most important link between the left and the right sides, and the injury caused a faulty connection. Peek was already four years of age when he learned to walk and was considered so severely mentally disabled that doctors suggested he be institutionalized.

But just like Michelle, Kim Peek recovered and developed in ways no one could have foreseen.

At around five years old, Peek learned to read, and whenever he finished a book he placed it front cover side down. His parents were astonished at the speed with which the house filled up with down-facing books. By then, Peek was also beginning to show a mind-boggling memory for detail, perhaps the best-ever documented in a human being. And he could read two pages in a book simultaneously, the left side with his left eye, and the right side with his right eye. It took him ten seconds to read one page; he could go through an entire book in one hour. His favorite pastime was going to the public library, where he would read eight books a day.

Basically, he remembered everything in the approximately twelve thousand books he had read. In his head, he kept an unimaginable amount of facts of varying degrees of importance; from Shakespeare, to facts about the British royal family, to the complete list of American zip codes. If anyone deserves to be called "the human Google," it's Kim Peek.

As with Michelle Mack, Peek could also immediately tell which weekday a date corresponded to, be they several decades in the future or in the past. People often walked up to Peek and told him their date of birth and asked him what day it was. Not only did he immediately give them the correct answer—"You were born on a Sunday"—but he could also add, "You will turn eighty on a Friday."

Kim Peek's abilities were so unique that he has been called "Kim-puter" and "megasavant," but things were far from simple for him in life. He was very awkward in social situations, and he was hardly able to dress himself. He tested quite a bit below average on IQ tests despite

16

his extraordinary memory. Peek was always generous and volunteered his time whenever neuroscientists asked to conduct studies on him, and his unique case has provided important clues to how memory works. It is now believed that Peek's outsize memory was a result of his brain's halves lacking contact and their inability to balance each other out.

THE BRAIN'S PROGRAMS CAN BE REWRITTEN

There are similarities as well as differences between Kim Peek and Michelle Mack. In Michelle's case, the connection was not absent; half her brain was simply not there. But the missing half of the brain might very well have had the same effect as a bad link between two existing brain halves, allowing certain abilities to grow uncontrollably and giving rise to exceptional qualities.

Kim Peek and Michelle Mack are perhaps the best examples of neuroplasticity—the brain's superb ability to reorganize itself—and there's no longer any doubt that the brain's structure and operating mode is changeable. Not only for Michelle Mack and Kim Peek, but also for you and me.

But why devote so much time to the story above in a book about the effects of exercise and athletic training on the brain? The reason is very simple: it is important to show that the brain *can* change, because not everyone is aware of this. The next question, then, is what creates this change? This is how we end up on the topic of physical activity and working out.

More like modeling clay than china

In the study of neuroplasticity, it has been shown that there are few things as effective in making the brain changeable—that is, neuroplastic— as being physically active. It also appears that the activity need not last an especially long time. In fact, only twenty to thirty minutes of physical activity are enough to affect neuroplasticity.

One of the mechanisms that converts your running steps to a changeable brain involves an amino acid called *gamma aminobutyric acid* (GABA). GABA acts like a brake on the brain, inhibiting activity and making sure nothing changes. But GABA's influence ebbs when you become physically active, because exercise removes GABA's block against change, thus making the brain more flexible and better at reorganizing itself. If we consider the brain from a more-like-modeling-clay-than-china perspective, the change in GABA activity makes the clay softer and more malleable.

The brain of a person who exercises becomes more like a child's, and GABA is involved in that process.

Hopefully, you have now realized how changeable the brain is, and that exercise and training play a big role in this change since they can modify and streamline our brain's programs. Physical activity produces results in many different areas, and we will now look a bit more closely at those areas, specifically at the impact training has on our mental functions. We'll start with what afflicts many people today: stress and anxiety.

DO WE ONLY USE 10 PERCENT OF OUR BRAIN?

It's time to put to rest the myth that we only use 10 percent of our brain. Of course, as you read that last sentence, it's not entirely unreasonable that you were using only 10 percent of your brain. It's also not impossible that you may only use 10 percent of your brain when you go for a bike ride (though not necessarily the same 10 percent you use when you're reading). In actuality, we do work our entire brain—just different parts of it, depending on what we're up to.

Today, we know that electrical activity and the use of glucose and oxygen—the brain's main fuels—is a continuous process in the brain. This means it is always active; no area remains idle in a healthy brain. The brain would never allow 90 percent of its capacity to stay dormant. Considering our brain's phenomenal ability to move different functions around—just think back to Michelle Mack—it would quickly put any quiet area to good use.

The "10 percent use" is obviously a myth, too, when accounting for our brain's energy consumption. The brain devours a substantial amount of energy—about 20 percent of all energy required by the body—even though the brain only makes up 2 percent of our body's total weight. This means that it spends more than ten times the energy per kilogram than the rest of the body. From an evolutionary standpoint, such an energy-draining organ wouldn't have been permitted to grow, were it unnecessary. The cost of a large brain is to consume more food, and with that there is a need to spend more time and energy to seek out this food. If the brain were indeed 90 percent inactive, then the time and energy expended would be a huge misuse of resources.

Compared to other species, it's clear that such waste would not have survived long on the path of natural selection.

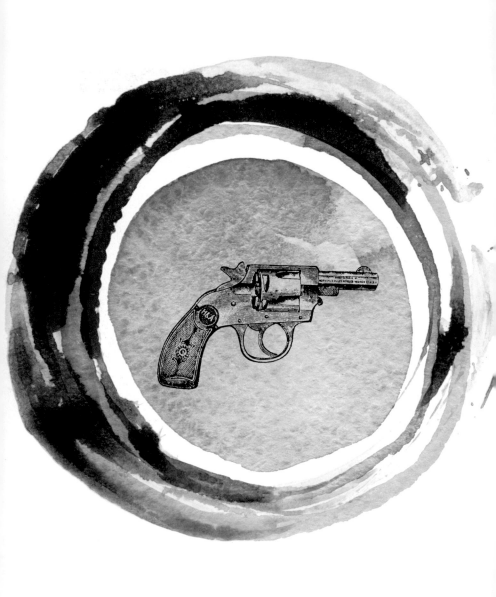

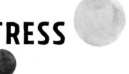

2. RUN AWAY FROM STRESS

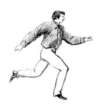

Whenever we feel stressed out, it's a sign that our brain is pumping out stress hormones. If sustained over months and years, those hormones can ruin our health and turn us into nervous wrecks.

ĐANIEL GOLEMAN

“The stress begins as soon as I open my eyes in the morning. Earlier than that, actually, because it is often stress that wakes me up. It feels like my brain is racing twenty-four-seven. I spend the entire day thinking about what I should do, and in the evening the anxiety continues to grind me, without any real reason for it.

“I live a hectic life. I do enjoy my job as a business attorney, but I wish it weren’t so time-consuming. I have a lot going on outside of work, too. I have two small children, so I have a perpetual guilty conscience because I’m not always on time to pick them up from day care; then there’s everything else that needs to be planned. Sometimes it seems as though life is just a round of logistics. But even though I have a lot to do at home and at work, I know I would have time for it all if I didn’t stress about it so much. The stress stops me, and I feel completely blocked.

“The stress has increased lately—either that or I’m less able to handle it. I have memory lapses, and I have become more and more absent-minded. I forgot my laptop in a restaurant after lunch, and it wasn’t until I got back to the office that I realized I had left it behind. It was sheer luck that I found it still there. This kind of thing has never happened before.

“The other day, I was on the bus and it was packed; suddenly I found it hard to breathe and had such a feeling of anxiety that I almost panicked.

RUN AWAY FROM STRESS

I ended up getting off a few stops early and walking the rest of the way. That has never happened before, either."

I met with this thirty-seven-year-old man in an outpatient psychiatric clinic. He told me how he had been feeling lately. He was a bit apprehensive to begin with and tried to downplay his problems as though he were ashamed, but eventually he became more open. The level of stress he had been experiencing over several years had gotten worse over time. He had trouble sleeping, and he got irritated over the slightest thing. He had been hiding his angst carefully from his surroundings. This man, married with two children, with a good job and a big apartment . . . what did he have to be unhappy about? All the outward signs of a successful life were there—but still, something was not right.

After almost an hour of talking, I explained to him that he seemed to have been under a great amount of pressure over a prolonged stretch of time, and that his symptoms—deteriorating memory, trouble sleeping, and the panic attack—most likely had their roots in this stress. He could consider antidepressant medication, but he was not interested in taking drugs. He asked if there were other options. I explained to him that talk therapy is usually effective, and that he should also begin an exercise program by taking up running. That sounded odd to him. "Medication and therapy—that's one thing, but running? How can that help with stress?"

It's safe to say that he is not alone in going through these problems. According to the American Psychological Association, 72 percent of all adult Americans experience recurring periods of high stress, and 42 percent suffer from insomnia as a result. Just like my thirty-seven-year-old patient, most of them are aware that medication and therapy are two methods of treating intense stress. And just like him, many don't know that maybe the most efficient treatment is what this book is all about: physical activity. In fact, exercise and training have shown impressive results in treating and preventing stress. I will now explain why this is the case, and how you, too, can go ahead and literally run away from stress and anxiety.

STRESS FULFILLS A FUNCTION

A good way to start coping with stress is to understand what stress is, and what function it fulfills. In your body, you have what is called the *HPA-axis*. The HPA-axis is located deep inside the brain, in the part called the *hypothalamus gland* (the *H* in HPA). When the brain detects something that it perceives as a threat, like someone screaming at you, the hypothalamus sends a signal to the pituitary gland (the *P* in HPA) in the brain. The pituitary reacts to the signal by sending out a hormone that goes into your bloodstream and over to your adrenal glands (the *A* in HPA). They, in turn, react by releasing the stress hormone cortisol, which makes the heart beat faster and harder. All this happens extremely fast; it only takes a second or so to go from you registering the shouting person, to the raised cortisol levels in the blood, to your increased heart rate.

Imagine that you're standing in front of a large group of colleagues, and you're about to do a presentation on a project that you've worked long and hard on. You feel your heart beat faster, and your mouth is dry even though you've just had a glass of water. You wonder if anyone notices that your hand is trembling slightly and that the notes you're holding are shaking a little. What is happening is your HPA-axis has started to rev up, and cortisol levels in your blood are rising. Your body interprets the situation as if it were confronted by danger, despite the fact that your coworkers are hardly a threat to your life. What begins in your body is a powerful set of biological mechanisms that has been maintained over millions of years of evolution. It has now become a matter of fight-or-flight for your body, even though in this case the "fight" means to give a good presentation and not to fend off a physical attack by your colleagues. However, from a purely biological standpoint, there is no doubt about it: your body is preparing itself for battle.

Rising levels of cortisol put both body and brain on high alert. Muscles need more blood when you're getting ready to fight or run for your life, so your heart beats faster and harder—an increased heart rate. Your brain becomes focused and sensitized to the smallest change. If you hear so much as a cough in your audience, you'll react to the sound at lightning speed.

So, stress fulfills a function. It makes you sharper and more focused, and while this is generally a good thing, the reaction can become far too intense for some. Instead of becoming more focused, they'll have trouble thinking clearly. They experience a loss of control and feel terrible distress. For them, the HPA-axis seems to be spinning out of control.

Amygdala—the stress trigger

But let's backtrack a bit to see where stress actually starts. The "warning" that your colleagues may constitute a danger doesn't come from the HPA-axis, but from its engine—*the amygdala*. The amygdala is a part of the brain the size of an almond, situated deep inside the temporal lobe. You have two amygdalae, one for each half of the brain. The amygdala has been preserved through evolution and is a feature of the brain that we share with many mammals. The reason for its continued presence through time is that it is incredibly important for the survival of our species, as well as that of others. And there's nothing very remarkable about that. If anything increases your chances of survival, it's having an effective alarm system that is good at signaling a dangerous situation so you can run away. That's just what the amygdala does.

The amygdala exhibits a singular property in the biological interplay of stress alarm activation. Not only does it trigger the stress function, it can also be triggered by it. Sound complicated? Here's how it happens: the amygdala signals danger, and this leads to elevated cortisol levels, which in turn activate the amygdala even *more*. The stress feeds on itself in a vicious circle.

If the amygdala is left to rev up the HPA-axis uncontrollably, sooner or later you will experience a full-fledged panic attack. Aside from being extremely unpleasant, a panic attack is never a good thing because the afflicted person often behaves irrationally. For our ancestors, panic was not compatible with survival when they came face-to-face with a threatening animal out in the savanna. However, what did increase their chances of survival was keeping a cool head and thinking clearly despite imminent danger.

The body has several built-in brake pedals to slow down the stress response, preventing it from going haywire and bringing on a panic attack. One of these is the hippocampus, which, though associated with the memory center, isn't just central to our ability to create memories; it also works like a brake so we don't overreact emotionally. The hippocampus can arrest the stress response, functioning like a counterweight to the amygdala's stress trigger. This happens continuously in your brain, and not just during stressful situations. There's always a balance between the amygdala and the hippocampus, each one pulling the other in opposite directions. The amygdala puts the pedal to the metal, while the hippocampus stands on the brakes.

The anxiety subsides

Let's get back to your presentation, which is now over, so you can take a breather. It doesn't look like your colleagues noticed your nervousness. Nobody even seems to have had an inkling of what felt like a chaotic storm raging inside you.

Your stress response decreases. Your body and brain lower their guard, as there no longer seems to be any threat. The amygdala's activities settle down, and cortisol levels drop. Your body lays down its weapons and backs off. You feel calmer.

It's important that cortisol levels fall as soon as the stressful situation blows over. A surge of cortisol is useful in a serious situation—you need that extra energy to fight or take flight—but walking around with elevated cortisol for an extended period is not a good thing. Too much of this stress hormone can in fact be a poison for the brain cells in the hippocampus, since they can die off from exposure to too much cortisol.

Over time—we're talking months and years here—an excess of cortisol is believed to make the hippocampus shrink in size.

Putting it mildly, this is not good news, because it can lead to memory problems. After all, the hippocampus is the brain's memory center, and many who experience prolonged elevated stress response, like my patient at the beginning of the chapter, experience worsening short-term memory. Some who have suffered from longtime high stress have difficulty finding words, while others forget places. The latter is more likely to occur because the hippocampus is also involved in spatial navigation.

Stress that creates stress

What is perhaps worse than forgetfulness is that a shrinking hippocampus becomes an increasingly weaker brake for the stress response. The hippocampus' stress brake gets worn down if the amygdala—the stress trigger—works overtime. The stress response begins to take on a life of its own when the hippocampus can no longer restrain the effects of the amygdala. The amygdala—the gas pedal—speeds up while the hippocampus—the brake—shrinks and becomes less able to slow things down. At this point we enter a vicious circle where stress creates more stress. This is exactly what can happen when there are drawn-out, or chronic, periods of stress: it can literally lead to the brain breaking down. When the brains of people suffering from high stress and anxiety were examined, it was found that their hippocampi were in fact a bit smaller than average, probably due to being slowly eroded by cortisol.

A BODY THAT IS PHYSICALLY FIT COPES BETTER WITH STRESS

It is an irrefutably good idea to attempt to curtail the effect of cortisol on the brain if you wish to get a better handle on stress. This is where exercise enters the picture. If you go for a run or a bike ride, or are otherwise active, cortisol levels will increase over the duration of the activity. This is because physical exertion is a type of stress on the body: your muscles need more energy and oxygen to work properly, so your heart will beat faster and harder to increase blood flow. Heart rate and blood pressure rise. The effects of cortisol in this case are not only normal; they're crucial for you to perform physically. But your body doesn't require the same stress response after your training session is over, so cortisol levels drop, in fact falling to below where they were before you had started running. If you keep up a regular running schedule, your cortisol will increase less and less during each successive running session and fall more and more every time you're done.

Now comes the real interesting part: if you continue to exercise regularly, your level of cortisol will increase less and less, even when you are under stress from reasons other than training. Your body's stress response, whether it be exercise or work-related, will improve as you become more physically fit. In a nutshell, training teaches the body to not overreact to stress.

Usually, the effect is unmistakable. Maybe you've noticed, as I have, that you're less sensitive to stress during times of intense training. You might go through a highly charged, busy workday, but when you think back on it later you'll notice that you hardly felt any stress. Often this cannot be explained away with a simple "I'm feeling a bit better overall" because you've exercised; instead it is the result of having strengthened your body's tolerance to stress through physical activity.

EXERCISE CALMS THE STRESS RESPONSE

The Montreal Imaging Stress Test (MIST) demonstrates how we react to stress. This is a computer-generated, timed test in which test subjects are asked to perform head math and mark their answers on the monitor. The result, whether right or wrong, is given immediately after each question.

Before the test, participants are informed that the average tester answered 80 to 90 percent of the questions correctly. When the test

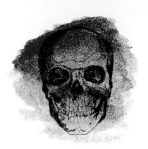

CORTISOL, THE "DEATH HORMONE"

Cortisol is sometimes referred to as the "death hormone," since we know that high levels of cortisol in the blood is damaging to the hippocampus, among other things. This moniker is unnecessarily harsh because the sole purpose of cortisol is not to break down the brain and cause damage; it has many important responsibilities. The trouble is that our stress response, starting with cortisol, has not evolved to contend with today's longer and higher-stress lifestyle.

In the environment from which human beings evolved—the savanna—stress was typically felt in short bursts. In a threatening situation, our ancestors could choose between going on the attack or running away. They didn't stay put, day after day, in front of an animal that wanted to eat them. In such situations, cortisol was a mobilizing force that gave us the strength to react.

Today, most of us don't have to worry about getting eaten or killed. However, stress brought on by work deadlines, bills to pay, and house repairs is not short-term, but persistent. When you worry about rising interests and pickup times at day care, the same response is activated as if you were standing in front of a hungry lion, except the reaction to the lion would be more intense. You run away from the lion—or get eaten by it—and the stress is gone. Fretting about your mortgage won't literally kill you, of course, but it will produce constant high levels of cortisol, which may beat up your brain in the end.

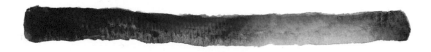

begins, the computer will only register 20 to 45 percent of the answers as correct, regardless of whether the subjects are right or wrong. During the test, it is revealed that the test subjects are indeed scoring well below average. Naturally, this is extremely aggravating, which is the intent of the exercise. It's not unusual for participants drop out of the test and leave in frustration.

The stress elevates blood pressure and increases the stress hormone cortisol, which is what the exercise is supposed to do. In other words, it's the stress reaction that is being studied with the MIST test, not how good testers are at mental arithmetic. So why am I telling you about this annoying test? Because it reveals the amazing impact exercise has on stress. Scientists asked a group of healthy subjects to ride a bike for thirty minutes before they took the test while another group performed gentle exercises without raising their heart rate. Afterwards, cortisol levels were lower in the testers who had biked, because they didn't react with as strong a stress response as the others. The result was the same, whether the participants were physically fit or not. Training calms the stress response, regardless of your physical condition.

It was also noted that the level of activity in the hippocampus (the part of the brain that acts like a brake on the stress response) was higher in the test subjects who had cycled. The entire HPA-axis was more subdued. The fact is that exercise and physical training is truly a gift for the hippocampus. On the whole, it seems like there's nothing more beneficial for the hippocampus than being active. As you will read in the chapter called *Jog your memory*, new cells are created in the hippocampus if you train regularly.

Allow your higher cognitive functions to nip anxiety in the bud

So the hippocampus acts like a brake on the stress response, brakes that are reinforced by physical training. But the hippocampus is not the only brake in your brain. The frontal lobe, which sits behind the forehead, can also inhibit the stress response. The frontal lobe, especially its anterior

Your body's stress response improves as you become more physically fit. Exercise teaches your body not to overreact to stress.

(front) part called the *prefrontal cortex*, is the seat of your higher cognitive functions. The ability to check/withhold impulses and abstract and analytical thought are situated here. During stress, the frontal lobe plays a central role in protecting you from overreacting emotionally and acting irrationally.

When the thought "Uh-oh, we're gonna crash!" hits you during a sudden bout of turbulence on a plane, it's the amygdala, quick as a flash, that puts your body on red alert—you're in fight-or-flight mode, with a racing heart, a surge of anxiety, or even a panic attack. The frontal lobe cools those feelings down with logic: "It was only an air pocket, and I've had this happen before. We didn't crash then, so why would we crash now?"

There is a constant tug-of-war going on between the amygdala and the frontal lobe, and not only during stressful times. Just like there's a balance between the amygdala and the hippocampus, there is a balance between the amygdala and the frontal lobe, and it can differ from person to person.

The reason some people are more susceptible to anxiety depends to a high degree on their amygdala signaling fear when there's no cause for it, while their frontal lobe is unable to push back and inhibit this predilection. Consequently, those people tend to see danger and potential catastrophes everywhere and walk around in a constant state of stress and foreboding.

Stress shrinks the thinking brain

Stress doesn't just shrink the hippocampus; it seems to have an identical effect on the frontal lobe. Indeed, parts of the frontal lobe are smaller in individuals with very anxious personalities. It could almost be considered as adding insult to injury! The longer the stress continues, the more the brain feeds on itself, and the worse the brakes work. Those suffering from chronic stress are most in need of their hippocampus and the frontal lobe, which don't function optimally for them.

When the amygdala sounds the alarm at every turn and the frontal lobe is unable to balance this out, we start to overreact to stuff that seems trivial. "When I said good morning to my boss this morning, she answered me a bit tersely. She probably doesn't like me. I must have done something wrong. I'm useless and I'll probably get fired soon." If the frontal lobe had stepped in properly, it would have helped gauge the situation more clearly: "My boss might have been a bit crabby this morning, but who isn't sometimes? Maybe she didn't sleep well."

When the frontal lobe becomes more active, we seem to become calmer and less stressed, and it becomes easier to withstand the anxiety generated by the amygdala. It has been possible to increase this activity by using magnetic field stimulation on the frontal lobe, simmering down the whole stress response.

In other words, strengthening the frontal lobe—the "thinking" part of the brain—is crucial if you want to put a damper on stress. Since this is a book about how exercise affects your brain, you might have already figured out that physical activity will strengthen your frontal lobe as well as your hippocampus. In fact, the frontal lobe and the hippocampus are the two areas of the brain that are helped the most when you move your body.

What effect does training have on the frontal lobe?

How does the frontal lobe become strong when you train? Well, in lots of ways! The frontal lobe receives more blood and works better as soon as you exercise, because blood flow in the brain increases when you're physically active. Over the long term, new blood vessels are created in the frontal lobe, improving the supply of blood and oxygen while at the same time removing more waste products.

Increased blood flow and new blood vessels are just the beginning. Today, we know that regular physical activity creates a closer connection between the frontal lobe and the amygdala, which enables the frontal lobe to control the amygdala more effectively—much like a teacher has a better grip on a class when he or she is present in the classroom, instead of trying to oversee things from another location.

Not only that, the frontal lobe also shows some long-term growth thanks to regular physical activity, a finding that surprised many in the field. It is a proven discovery, not merely an assumption. When the sizes of the frontal lobes of healthy adults were measured at regular intervals as they took hour-long walks, the measurements indicated that the brain's outer covering, the cerebral cortex, seemed to develop further. It seems incredible that we can measure how our frontal lobe can get bigger just by taking walks!

Everybody knows that working out leads to bigger muscles, but you probably weren't aware that it also makes the more sophisticated part of the brain—the part that separates us from other animals—develop further. However, there is a catch: you must hang in there, continually exercising, and never give up! The frontal lobe won't acquire more favorable conditions to better control the amygdala overnight; it could take months. Even if training alleviates stress straight away, there's all the more reason to persevere.

You won't appreciate the full benefits on your general well-being and stress tolerance until after a few months of sustained exercise. But you will notice them in many ways because the effects of lowered activity of the brain's stress response go much deeper than simply being able to handle stress better. Research also indicates that a person's self-confidence gets a boost when activity in the brain's stress response area—the HPA-axis—is lowered. Self-confidence is a trait that is linked to stress and anxiety, among other things.

Are medications too effective?

There are medications available for treating stress and anxiety that provide quick relief. You've probably heard of some, if not all of them: Diazepam,

Oxazepam, Rohypnol, and Xanax. The problem with these drugs is not that they are ineffective, since stress and anxiety often subside soon after the drugs have been ingested. Rather, the issue is that they work *too* well.

The brain is programmed to seek out stress relief, which is why pills that ensure immediate shelter from anxiety and that bestow a sense of calm are enormously tempting. The risk is that your brain will scream for these medications once you've tried them once. Furthermore, the brain tends to adapt quickly, so after only a short course of treatment, brain chemistry can change, and what provided effective relief at first is no longer enough. The dose needs to be increased to deliver the same effect, at which point you run the risk of becoming addicted.

Besides the aforementioned drugs, there is another substance that has an amazing ability to turn off feelings of stress and anxiety, and it carries with it a major risk of dependency. That substance is alcohol. Alcohol is extremely effective at quickly lowering the stress response. In fact, there are few, if any, other substances that are comparable to alcohol's power to provide relief from stress and anxiety. Anyone who has ever drunk wine or spirits when he or she felt anxious knows exactly what I'm talking about—a few minutes is all it takes for all the worry to vanish.

Alcohol and anxiolytic drugs have such similar effects that many anxiolytics reproduce "dry drunk" syndrome in people. Their common denominator is that they both target the same system in the brain—the GABA.

Your stress extinguisher

Gamma-aminobutyric acid (GABA) is an amino acid whose purpose is to calm the brain and act as a fire extinguisher to enable brain cells to suppress their activities. Once the brain's activities are calmed, feelings of stress disappear. Consequently, GABA activation provides quick and effective stress relief, exactly as if you were drinking alcohol or taking anxiolytics.

What is cool about GABA is that it isn't just activated by alcohol and pills; it's also activated by movement (i.e., exercise). Walking yields a

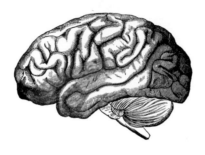

ANATOMY OF STRESS

There is a physical connection through several nerve pathways between the frontal lobe and the amygdala. Today, we believe that the better the pathways are at transmitting information, the better the frontal lobe acts as a damper on the amygdala to suppress feelings of stress and anxiety.

We can look at the nerve pathways as stress and anxiety's true anatomy, and the physical coupling of your rational, thinking brain and your reptilian brain. The magnitude of anxiety and stress problems appears to be associated with how thick these pathways are. Thick nerve paths are better at transmitting signals between the different areas of the brain, and a thick pathway means that the frontal lobe is more effective at controlling the amygdala. In fact, current modern medical technology allows us to measure the thickness of the neural pathways. One of the most significant pathways between the amygdala and the frontal lobe is called *uncinate fasciculus* (UF), which measures between 4 and 5 cm (1.57 to 1.96 inches) in length. Upon examining people suffering from what is commonly called *Generalized Anxiety Disorder* (GAD), it has been shown that their UP path is less efficient at transmitting signals. In all likelihood, this means that their frontal lobe has less ability to act as a brake on the amygdala, which leads to anxiety and stress.

certain effect, but the best results come from running or biking. Today we know that sustained physical exertion causes GABA activity to ramp up, especially in areas of the brain situated below the cerebral cortex. It's from this area that a lot of stress originates. That GABA activity increases there as well means that training strikes at the very heart of the stress.

"Nanny neurons"

It is probably GABA that causes the paradox of training's effect on the brain. As you will see in the upcoming chapter *Jog your memory*, exercise leads to the creation of new brain cells, and new brain cells are like new people (i.e., small children) in that they are extremely active. To get a three-year-old to sit calmly is just about impossible. It's the same for young brain cells, which are always active and which like to send signals to other cells without any prompting from their surroundings. They do as they please. This might seem kind of cute, but easily revved-up brain cells are bad news from the standpoint of stress because they can create feelings of anxiety. Anyone who experiences a lot of stress and anxiety might prefer to have calm brain cells that don't fire off at will.

What is remarkable is that while training causes new, hyper-active cells to form, which should bring about more stress and anxiety, you become calm instead. This is probably because some of the new cells created through exercise are GABA cells, which, instead of going out of control, help to inhibit overactivity in new-born cells.

In popular science articles, these GABA cells are sometimes called *nanny neurons,* which suggests that their role is to calm other young brain cells. The soothing influence of those nanny neurons on their environment causes the entire brain to settle down. It appears that if you work out, you can create more nanny neurons to effectively inhibit activity—and therefore stress levels—in the brain. "And where do these nanny neurons form?" you may ask yourself.

Animal testing has shown that they form primarily in an area of the hippocampus that is important in regulating emotions and inhibiting anxiety. Even there, exercise takes aim at the heart of stress and anxiety.

YOUR MUSCLES ARE A STRESS TREATMENT PLANT

Scientists genetically manipulated some mice so they were born with more developed muscles, and they seemed to be more or less immune to stress. Each attempt to worry the animals with bright lights and loud noises failed—they appeared to have nerves of steel. What was in the muscles that protected the mice from stress? Well, there is something in muscles that neutralizes a metabolite called *kynurenine*, which is caused by stress.

The stress metabolite kynurenine can be dangerous for the brain, but with assistance from the muscles it is neutralized and thus prevented from entering the brain. It's very likely that this helped make the mice completely impervious to stress. The same mechanism for neutralizing the stress metabolite is present in human muscles, as well. This suggests that muscles are able to work as a type of treatment plant to remove damaging stress triggers. In the same way that the liver purifies blood by removing toxic substances, muscles protect the brain.

If muscles can neutralize an important stress substance, then it's easy to infer that we could become better at dealing with stress by training our muscles. While a lot points to that conclusion since the muscled mice appeared resistant to stress, we don't have firm answers yet as to how big the impact would be on us humans.

Even strength is good for stress

The experiment with the muscled mice is even more exciting because it is one of the first instances where it has been possible to show how strength training by itself can be good for combating stress. Scientists

Anxiety is the price we pay for our intelligence.

WHY DO WE WORRY?

The body's built-in stress and anxiety mechanisms are there to increase our chances for survival. At the same time, living and surviving in today's society is easier than it was in any other time in history. Most of us don't need to worry about encountering danger, not having enough food, or not having a roof over our head, so it might seem contradictory that we still experience such high levels of stress and anxiety. We should all be walking around, calm and serene. Why aren't we?

You'll find the answer in our past. Picture two groups of your ancestors on the savanna. One group is contented, taking it easy, scratching themselves between their toes, and feeling that everything will turn out just fine. *"Mañana, mañana."* The other group is dissatisfied and worried. "Do we have enough to eat? What if the weather turns bad? We may not find any more zebras or antelopes to hunt—let's go out and fill the larder to be on the safe side."

Which group do you think had the biggest odds of living a long life? I'd place my bet on the anxious group for sure. The fact that we experience anxiety and stress has helped us a great deal in planning for the future, and it has increased our chances of survival. It is not nature playing a nasty prank on us when we feel stressed out and anxious; it's a survival mechanism that allowed our ancestors to forge ahead. This mechanism doesn't fit our present-day life very well, but it's still there in us whether we like it or not. And it does explain why training is so beneficial in combating stress and anxiety: being physically active back in the day meant hunting for food or running away from danger—in other words, doing something to survive. So when we run on the treadmill, our brain interprets this as an activity that increases our chance of survival, which in turn relieves our stress and anxiety.

A more philosophical spin would be to assert that our anxiety is the direct outcome of our intelligence. Having the ability to plan the future and to think of how it *might* turn out enables us to worry about things we'd prefer to avoid. That is how humans are unique. Our stress response can start now if we begin to brood about what *could* happen at work next week, without it being a real threat at this very moment. The ability to anticipate danger also means that we can plan on how to avoid it and worry about it before it becomes a fait accompli. Anxiety is the price we pay for our intelligence.

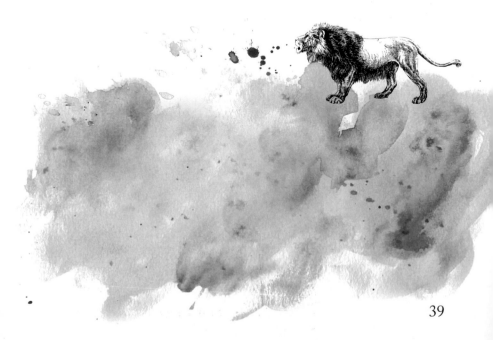

have often focused their attention on the effects of aerobic training, but in this case, it's all about our *muscles'* stress-busting potential. So, can we conclude from these findings that we should rely on strength training alone to protect ourselves against stress? No, absolutely not. Even taking this into account, it's better to vary the type of physical activity you engage in and incorporate both strength and cardiovascular training.

TACKLE ANXIETY FROM DIFFERENT SIDES

Are you beginning to see why training is extremely good for anyone suffering from stress and anxiety? It attacks the problem from several sides! Cortisol levels fall after each training session and won't rise as much the next time. The hippocampus and the frontal lobe—the stress response's brake pedals—strengthen and become more efficient at inhibiting the amygdala/anxiety engine. Activity in the brain's GABA brake system is enhanced with more nanny neurons, and the muscles' ability to neutralize the stress substance increases. All this takes place simultaneously.

In reality, it's difficult to tease the different mechanisms apart and to figure out how much anxiety inhibition is due to, say, decreased cortisol levels and how much of it is because of GABA. But if we combine all the mechanisms and look at the end result—which is what is truly interesting, after all—there's no doubt that exercise and physical training are fantastic antidotes to stress, maybe even the very best!

Teenage angst no more

The number of teenagers seeking psychiatric help for stress and anxiety has risen steadily over the past few years. From a biological standpoint, teenage anxiety is nothing exceptional. The areas of the brain that dampen stress and anxiety, including the frontal lobe and prefrontal cortex, are the last to mature. They are not fully developed in

40

a teenager; in fact, they're not completely mature until about twenty-five years of age. However, areas that *create* stress, like the amygdala, are often fully developed in a seventeen-year-old. With the anxiety trigger in full working order while the anxiety inhibitor is not, the teenage years are a period rife with mood swings, impulsivity, and anxiety.

Still, exercise can have a huge impact even on teenagers' feelings of stress and anxiety. A study in Chile was conducted on two hundred healthy ninth-graders hailing from a vulnerable area of Santiago, the country's capital. Chile had only recently begun to suffer from western-style diseases such as diabetes and cardiovascular disease, and scientists wanted to see if it was possible to reverse that trend with lifestyle changes. They also wanted to check if regular training would influence the youth's well-being and self-confidence.

At the end of the ten-week program, the tests revealed that the training had not only produced great fitness results, but also improved the teenagers' confidence and sense of well-being. Furthermore, what stood out was the effect the program had on their stress and anxiety levels, which had fallen significantly. The teenagers felt much calmer, less anxious, and more self-confident.

Less stressed-out and less cynical

Do you think that the anxiety you feel has nothing to do with teenage angst? In a study to find out why some people have heart attacks, and how stress might be involved, over three thousand Finnish men were asked to answer questions about their lifestyle. A summary of the results showed that the men who exercised at least twice a week had fewer issues with stress and anxiety; this is the same pattern that had been found in Chile. Those who trained were also less prone to aggression and had a less cynical outlook on life.

So is this *solid proof* that physical activity lessens stress and anxiety? No. We don't know for sure if it was the training that made the Finnish men less stressed-out and worried. Maybe it's a case where individuals who are less worried train more. You must use caution when drawing conclusions if you're only looking at results from the Finnish and the Chilean studies. However, if you look at them together with all the other research that has been carried out, the picture becomes crystal clear: exercise has a dramatic impact on stress and anxiety throughout life, in both the young and the old.

STRESS'S DOMINANT PLACE IN THE BRAIN

It's easy to think of stress as purely negative, but of course things are not quite that simple; on the contrary, stress is essential to our ability to function. Before learning how to better handle stress and worry—through exercise and other means—you must understand how important stress is and what it does for us.

To find out how important something is, remove it. What would happen if we simply knocked out the stress response system? This was the question scientists sought to answer when they surgically removed the amygdala from a group of monkeys. They suspected that the surgery would interfere with the animals' ability to feel fear, so to explore this hypothesis they brought in some company that most people and animals feel very uncomfortable around—snakes.

Just like humans, monkeys normally have a deeply ingrained fear of snakes. But there was no trace of fear in the monkeys whose amygdalae had been removed—quite the contrary. Instead of keeping out of harm's way, they were almost too interested in the snakes, playing with them and swinging them around.

The woman who couldn't feel fear

The monkeys didn't seem to care at all about the risk they were being exposed to, but was it because they could no longer feel fear, or did they misunderstand the entire situation? Had the surgery damaged their brains and made them unable to understand what they were doing? Did they not think the snakes were dangerous? It would have been incontestably difficult to ask monkeys how they perceived the situation; it would have been far simpler to study people without amygdalae, but such individuals are few and far between.

This being the case, American scientists jumped at the chance to learn more about the amygdala and its stress response when they encountered a forty-four-year-old mother who suffered from Urbach-Wiethe disease, an extremely rare genetic disease. Less than four hundred cases have been reported since it first became known in the 1920s. This condition causes destruction in parts of the brain, including the temporal lobe (where the amygdala is situated), which for some reason is especially vulnerable. In this woman's case, only her amygdalae—one in each side of her brain—were affected.

This woman, who was of normal intelligence despite her condition, willingly took part in a series of tests to see if the absence of amygdala affected her sense of fear. The scientists brought her to a pet store to gauge her reaction to snakes, like they had done with the monkeys. They also tested her reaction to spiders. Before this field trip, the woman had asserted that she had always had an aversion to snakes and spiders. Even so, she walked right up to the terrarium, fascinated by a collection of very large snakes. They were lifted out so that she could pet them, and according to the staff she didn't hesitate for a second to stroke them, even though she had been warned that the snakes could bite. The researchers asked the woman to grade her fear on a ten-point scale, zero representing no fear at all, and ten being most fearful. Playing with large, potentially life-threatening reptiles was rated a two.

The same thing happened when she was left to pet large, hairy tarantulas. The store's staff explained that she became almost obsessed with touching the animals without any precaution. She continued to play with them until the staff interrupted and stopped her because she ran the risk of being bitten and the situation wasn't considered safe anymore. It didn't seem to bother her in the least that this spider was especially aggressive and dangerous. As a matter of fact, she was almost careless with it in a way that was reminiscent of how the monkeys had played with the snakes.

It's very tempting to assume that the reason for her recklessness was her destroyed amygdalae. But before we reach this conclusion, it would be prudent, as in the case of the monkeys, to speculate whether there could have been another cause. Maybe it was only a fear of animals—even if those animals were the kind we tend to feel most anxious around—that had been affected. Perhaps she would feel frightened if confronted by something else? The next step was to have her watch disturbing scenes from horror films such as *The Shining*, *The Ring*, and *The Blair Witch Project*, movies that typically spook most people out. To ensure that the clips were creepy enough, they were first shown to a group of test subjects who were asked to rate their scariness on a scale of one to ten. Most of the clips scored between six and seven.

But those same film clips failed to arouse any fear in the woman, who gave them a score of zero. Oddly enough, however, she seemed interested in the films and thought they looked exciting. She even asked for the title of one of them so she could rent it and finish watching the movie at home.

Aside from participating in experiments featuring scary animals and horror films, the woman was followed for several years. The picture that emerged was clear: it appeared that she had become utterly fearless after her amygdalae were destroyed. But no other feelings had been affected—she could be happy, elated, or sad, depending on the circumstances. While showing the film clips, the researchers saw clues that other feelings were intact. The creepy clips were interspersed with excerpts from comedies and dramas to provoke other feelings besides fear. The woman reacted normally when watching these: she laughed at comedic moments and expressed sadness while watching a scene featuring an abandoned child. The absence of working amygdalae had not made her apathetic or emotionally disengaged to the point of not being able to feel anything. It had only taken away her ability to feel fear.

It's almost enough to make one jealous! Imagine never having to be afraid or worried, and being able to face most things in life without a care in the world. However, it wasn't so easy for our test subject. Her inability to feel fright had severe repercussions, because she put herself into dangerous situations several times; she had been robbed and threatened both with a knife and a gun. Normally these types of experiences would lead to anxiety, and most of us would be more careful and avoid areas where we've been accosted and robbed at knifepoint. However, she quickly got over those events and kept going without changing her behavior in the slightest. She lived in an economically depressed area plagued by drugs and violence, yet she went out late at night to dangerous places. Despite the unsafe environment, she did not seem to have learned to avoid perilous situations.

Our deepest fear

Was she completely immune to fear, then? No, because scientists eventually found something that made her completely freak out, and that was dyspnea—shortness of breath or choking. Inhaling carbon dioxide awakened a terror she was previously unable to feel. If you don't breathe in enough air, the level of carbon dioxide rises quickly in the body. It is actually the increase of carbon dioxide, and not the lack of oxygen, that the brain swiftly reacts to, since it interprets the inhalation of carbon dioxide as suffocation. This fear is probably more deeply rooted than any other type of dread. If you breathe in carbon dioxide, you will, sooner rather than later, be gripped by total panic. This is exactly what happened to the test subject, who for the first time in her life experienced such all-out terror that she screamed, shook, and gasped for air. Her brain alerted her to a life-threatening situation, and it did so without the amygdalae.

Later, when asked about her experience, the woman explained that the feeling was not only the most intense she'd ever had, it was also completely new to her. So why did she feel panic at the prospect of suffocation, but not when facing snakes, spiders, and horror movies? One possible explanation is that the amygdala is necessary for us to gauge external dangers, such as a snake or a person threatening us with a weapon, but not to internal threats. An external occurrence must be interpreted as such: the man in front of me with a knife is dangerous. On the other hand, the feeling of suffocation requires no explanation because that fear is deep-seated within us.

The amygdala takes charge

The examples with the monkeys and the woman illustrate the override function of the stress response in the brain. Moreover, they show the amygdala's role as a warning flag in the face of danger and as an engine of the stress response. The amygdala is extremely powerful and can very quickly switch the heart and body into action mode, leaving no room to think of long-term consequences. The brake pedals available to the brain—the hippocampus and the frontal lobe, for instance—that engage deliberation and forethought don't stand a chance in a truly dire situation. Quite simply, they are barreled over by the amygdala.

When we lived in the environment out of which we have evolved—the savanna—it was critical that the amygdala be forceful. It was vitally important to be able make lightning-quick decisions if we were threatened by an animal.

"Do I attack, or am I defenseless and need to run away from here?" In this type of situation, there's no time to weigh the pros and cons for too long, or it could be too late. Instead, it's important that the amygdala take charge and override the rest of the brain to be able to react immediately, either by attacking or scampering away.

This mechanism isn't needed as much in our current society, in which we're seldom faced with life-and-death situations that require quick decisions. Now there's the risk of the amygdala's power targeting something that isn't all that dangerous, to which we overreact emotionally. In the mid-1990s, the American psychologist Daniel Goleman coined the term *amygdala hijack*. This means an exaggerated emotional reaction, the result of the amygdala putting such strong emotional emphasis on an event that it's perceived as being a far worse threat than it objectively is. The amygdala hijacks the brain and forces the individual into fight-or-flight mode where he or she no longer reacts rationally.

It's not enough for a strong emotional reaction to qualify as amygdala hijacking; it also needs to happen quickly and leave you feeling remorseful afterwards. One of Goleman's prime examples was when the boxer Mike Tyson bit off Evander Holyfield's ear during a bout. Tyson acted fast—probably more like a reflex—and he seemed to have met the criteria for exhibiting remorse to the fullest. Aside from the embarrassment, that bite cost him millions of dollars in fines and legal fees. According to Daniel Goleman, this is a typical example of amygdala hijacking.

INCREASE STRESS TOLERANCE

When we realize how powerful the brain's amygdala and stress response are, we also come to understand why we can't remove stress completely from our lives, since it's far too deeply ingrained in the brain for that to be possible. We can certainly try to avoid the things that stress us out the most, but striving for a totally stress-free life would mean that you would have to move out into the wild and isolate yourself! Then you'd probably stress out because you'd be all alone!

Since it's impossible to eliminate all stress from life, a much better goal is to increase your tolerance to stress. That's exactly what physical activity does; it won't erase stress, but it'll help you handle it better. Regular exercise strengthens the brain's brake pedals, so it'll take a lot more for you to enter that fight-or-flight mode. Let's say that you get reprimanded at work for missing a deadline. If you're fit, the likelihood of you entering *panic mode*—with its quickening heart rate, rising blood pressure, and muddled thinking—is lessened. Training increases the chance that you'll be able to cope with such a situation and not overreact physically or psychologically.

I also want to say to those of you who think you're too stressed out to make time for regular training that it is precisely *you* who are most in need of physical exercise! And here's a tip for anyone who believes they have too much on their plate to train: not only will you feel better and less stressed out if you make time to exercise, but it will also be time well spent with regards to your job performance. I dare say that if you swap an hour at work for an hour's training from time to time, you'll get a lot more done during the rest of the day. At any rate, that's how it works for me.

Stress shows up on the scales

I have one ace left up my sleeve, just in case you're still not convinced that exercising is a good way to manage stress. What most motivates people to begin running or visiting the gym is *not* that it will make them healthy, feel good, or handle stress better. It is what they see in the mirror! More than anything, weight loss or developing an athletic body is what prompts most of us to become physically active. And I've got some good news here: if you increase your tolerance to stress by training, it will show up on the scales and in the mirror, too.

If you exchange a working hour, now and then, for an hour's physical training, you'll get much more done during the rest of the workday.

This is because the stress hormone cortisol prevents the body from burning fat. Having high levels of cortisol leads the body to store abdominal fat. Moreover, it increases appetite, especially for calorie-dense foods. If you're under a lot of stress and walk around with high cortisol levels, you'll risk adding more pounds around your waist and experiencing major sugar cravings. Handling your stress levels through exercise means that you lower your cortisol levels, which, over the long haul, can decrease your appetite and fat storing, increase fat burning, and show appreciable results on the scales and around your waist!

STRESS IS TRANSIENT—ANXIETY STICKS AROUND

You've probably experienced anxiety at one time or another—everybody does—but likely without knowing what it was. When patients ask me to explain what anxiety is, I usually say it is an overwhelming feeling of dread, of not having peace of mind, of feeling that something is wrong and that you would like to crawl out of your own skin.

It's not always easy to make the distinction between stress and anxiety, but it is commonly said that stress is a reaction to something that happens here and now and that is perceived as a threat. On the other hand, anxiety is worry connected to something that isn't a threat at present, or to something that has happened, or might possibly happen. When you are berated at work because of a mistake you've made, what you feel is stress. Anxiety is the tension you feel one week later, even if you're not at work and the incident is long past. Stress is transient, while anxiety stays around. Basically, it is the same stress response (i.e., the HPA-axis) causing both states of mind.

Is anxiety an illness, or does it fulfill a function? If we look at anxiety frankly, from a biological perspective, it is a feeling of fear and dread that follows an experience that we have perceived as a threat where there was none. The intensity of this lingering feeling can vary. Anxiety, just like stress, casts a wide net and can cover everything from being slightly uncomfortable to full-blown panic. Anxiety can come and go, as in the case of a panic attack, or lie low and simmer over time, as with generalized anxiety disorder. Anxiety can be brought on by traumatic memories, as with PTSD (Posttraumatic Stress Disorder), or flare up in social settings (social phobia). Although only a few anxiety disorders are officially recognized, in reality there are as many variations on anxiety as there are people.

But is anxiety dangerous? Many who have experienced intense anxiety due to panic attacks believe that it is. Some even fear that they are going to die. Many also think that they are alone in their plight. They are all wrong. Even if anxiety is unpleasant, it is neither dangerous nor rare. Your heart will not stop if you are anxious, even if it feels like it might. And the sufferer is *not* alone; anxiety is both a common and benign reaction that most of us experience to a different degree, and that at times can go completely overboard for some of us.

Unconscious fear

We can inquire about what causes anxiety. We know that sufferers have an overactive and easily triggered amygdala that signals danger without any threat being present; they see potential catastrophes on every street corner without being conscious of it. Individuals were tested by having pictures of angry and neutral faces shown during a time span of just two hundredths of a second. In the best-case scenario, people saw that it was a face but found it impossible to register the expression. Even though the face flashed too quickly for anybody to pick out a facial expression, anxiety-ridden people would react differently to the pictures.

TRAINING OR RELAXATION?

As you learn more about the research around how training affects stress, it becomes obvious that everybody, both children and adults, ought to engage in physical exercise in one form or another. It doesn't mean that you should disregard relaxation, meditation, mindfulness practices, or yoga, which might also be good. However, if you don't train, you might miss out on perhaps the most effective way to handle stress and anxiety. And if you have to choose between training and, for example, relaxation, training is always the better choice. If everybody just became more physically active—and I'm not talking about running a marathon—it would have mind-boggling consequences on the stress levels people are living with today. Fewer people would need psychiatric help and nearly everybody—whether they suffer from stress or not—would feel much better.

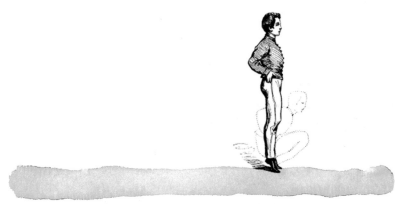

When scientists examined individuals' brains with MRI while they looked at the pictures of angry faces, the amygdalae of anxiety sufferers were visibly more easily activated. Moreover, the bigger the anxiety issue, the quicker the amygdalae were fired up by the angry faces, even though the viewer was not conscious of what he or she saw! However, for neutral facial expressions, which cannot be interpreted as a threat, there was no discernable difference between the amygdala's reaction in healthy people and that of those suffering from anxiety disorder. People suffering from high anxiety have an amygdala that's always in the starting blocks, ready to go and prepared to signal danger, and in so doing it activates the body's stress response.

Exercise your anxiety away

It's often difficult to separate stress from anxiety. After all, it's all part of the same system (including the HPA-axis and the amygdala), which is active in both stress and anxiety. Physical training, as you have seen earlier, has an amazing effect on stress, which is why training is also a great way to treat anxiety.

When American students suffering from anxiety drew lots to either walk or run for twenty minutes a few times a week over the course of two weeks—hardly a grueling training regimen either way—it showed that anxiety levels fell for both the walkers and the runners. The anxiety wasn't just lowered after the exercise, it stayed low over next twenty-four hours, and the effect lasted an entire week. Who experienced the highest impact on their anxiety levels? The runners did. More effort is obviously better if you wish to lower your anxiety.

This isn't surprising, if you think about it. Anxiety is caused by overactivity of the brain's stress response and an amygdala that signals danger where there is none. Training strengthens the brain's brake pedals against worry, and the frontal lobe and hippocampus become better at calming the amygdala, thereby preventing anxiety.

Anxiety—a learning problem

In principle, everyone would experience high anxiety if they were exposed to a life-threatening situation; on the other hand, not everyone becomes overwhelmed by anxiety when stepping onto a subway train. I once had a patient who suffered a severe panic attack, complete with a racing heart and trouble breathing, in the subway. Her terror was so strong that she was convinced she was going to die. If you've experienced this, you know that it'd be common to feel anxious about riding the subway again. That's what happened to this woman, who, since her attack, has chosen to travel exclusively by bus. It isn't that she didn't understand that subway cars aren't dangerous, it's that her brain misinterpreted the situation. The mechanisms that misread the event were so powerful that they overrode her "thinking brain."

The amygdala, as you have seen, is so powerful that it can overrule the brain. Moreover, it is excellent at making sure we remember threatening situations very well. If you've had a panic attack in the subway once, you will remember it very clearly. This is logical from the point of view of survival. We are programmed to distinctly remember what turned out to be unpleasant and/or dangerous so we can avoid it in the future. From an evolutionary perspective, it's not as critical to remember the five beautiful clearings in the woods as it is to remember where the wolf charged at us. Because of this, negative memories take precedence.

Memories that are connected to fear are so vivid that they can become a hindrance when you wish to treat anxiety disorders such as panic attacks. For anyone who has experienced a panic attack on a subway train, walking past a subway entrance can be enough to tell the amygdala to trigger the stress response and the HPA-axis. Even if this person eventually overcomes his or her fear and dares to ride the train again, it can take a long time before he or she feels okay or at peace doing so. The unpleasant memory is so strong that it blanks out all the memories of uneventful subway trips without panic attacks.

Considered this way, you can view anxiety disorders as a learned behavior problem. The brain can't learn that something is not dangerous. However, if it is programmed to clearly retain the memory of what is threatening, how can we ever be free of anxiety and worry? Well, the solution is to slowly and patiently build up new memories where, for example, a subway ride is not full of panic or apprehension. This is exactly what takes place during CBT (Cognitive Behavioral Therapy), during which a patient is gradually introduced to more of what causes his or her anxiety in order to relearn that it isn't dangerous. This memory slowly morphs from an anxiety-inducing misinterpretation to something the brain considers neutral and nonthreatening.

Increased heart rate doesn't have to mean anxiety

This leads us to another reason why training is so beneficial in treating anxiety. Heart rate and blood pressure increase in tandem with symptoms of high anxiety. The heart beats faster and harder, and the body goes into fight-or-flight mode, prepared for something negative to take place. But remember, the heart also beats faster and harder if you are out jogging, without your training session ending in some kind of unpleasant episode. Instead, you feel calm when the run is over, and you're rewarded with surges of endorphins and dopamine. Exercise teaches the brain that a raised heart rate and blood pressure don't mean anxiety and panic, but rather that positive feelings will ensue.

This is exactly what was observed in the anxiety-ridden American students who were asked to walk and run. Those who ran were no longer nervous about their heightened heart rate. When before they had equated a racing heart with an imminent anxiety attack, their body had since made the adjustment that an elevated rate was not a threat but the opposite—it could be a positive thing. This effect was not seen in those who walked—their brains still appeared to be misinterpreting the quicker heart rate as dangerous. This underscores the importance of moving more intensely if you wish to overcome anxiety and worry.

It was once believed that those experiencing a lot of anxiety and worry should avoid physical activity. Today we know that nothing could be further from the truth. However, I must warn that it's important to start out carefully if you have ever suffered a panic attack. Intense training can be risky, because it could be misinterpreted by the body as an impending crisis and cause an attack in someone who isn't ready. For that reason, it's better to start out slowly and ramp up the effort gradually.

Exercise is the opposite of stress

When you look closely at research on physical activity and stress, a clear pattern emerges: stress and physical training seem to have almost opposing effects on the brain. Increased stress (i.e., having high levels of the stress hormone cortisol) impedes brain cells' ability to communicate with one another, whereas training boosts that ability. Stress decreases the brain's ability to change (its plasticity), while training increases it. Higher stress applies the brake on the change from short-term memory to long-term memory, while training releases it, and so on. In area after area, it appears that stress and training yield the exact opposite effects. This literally makes exercise and physical activity an antidote to stress and anxiety!

TRAIN AND PREVENT PANIC ATTACKS

There are some who will do just about anything to help advance the cause of research. I would like to introduce the twelve bravest test subjects I know. They all agreed to receive an injection of the substance CCK4 (Cholecystokinin tetrapeptid 4). CCK4 has an extremely nasty side effect: it can bring on a panic attack, complete with breathing difficulties and a racing heart. The feeling is so strong that some believe they're going to die. This is what happened to six of the twelve participants: they broke out in a cold sweat, had trouble breathing, and were overcome by paralyzing fear, even though none of them had ever suffered panic attacks before.

This test was then repeated—amazingly, the test subjects agreed to volunteer again—but with a big difference: the participants exercised quite intensely (at 70 percent of maximum capacity) for thirty minutes prior to getting their CCK4 injection. At this point, something extraordinary happened: only one test subject experienced a panic attack. Evidently the training showed immediate results and decreased the likelihood of having such episodes.

Agreeing to be injected with a panic-inducing substance is undeniably brave, but another test group showed even more guts. This group had experienced panic attacks before and knew how horrible they could be. And yet they consented to go through yet another one, by administering CCK4. Despite only getting half a dose compared to the healthy group, nine people in the test group had a panic attack. But, as with the healthy group, the number of panic attacks declined when the test subjects were authorized to exercise beforehand. Only four out of the twelve subjects experienced a panic attack; furthermore, they felt that the event was less severe than those they had experienced before.

Thus, training has a preventive effect on panic attacks, both in prior sufferers and in those who have never experienced one. If exercise works on such severe cases of anxiety, it should definitely help with the "garden variety" anxiety that so many of us grapple with today.

THE RIGHT PRESCRIPTION TO RID YOURSELF OF STRESS AND ANXIETY

Realistically, which is the best way to train to rid yourself of stress and anxiety? Based on research, there is no custom program that specifies how intensely or how long you should move to lower your stress level and prevent anxiety; everyone responds differently to exercise, which is why no such systematic comparisons have been undertaken. However, even though there isn't one single, definite program that works for everyone, there are some concrete tips based on scientific research, that you can follow.

Focus on cardiovascular training at the outset. It appears that aerobic training is more beneficial than weight training from a stress-relief standpoint. Work out for at least twenty minutes; try to make it thirty to forty-five minutes if you have the stamina.

Make training into a habit because the results will only get better as you go along. It takes time before the hippocampus and the frontal lobe—two of the brain's stress brakes— become stronger.

Try to get your heart rate up at least two to three times a week. Your body will then learn that a faster heartbeat is not a cause for fear, but a state of being that brings about positive changes. This is especially important if you suffer from more serious anxiety problems and panic attacks.

Aim to reach the point of fatigue once a week—with interval training, for example. There are many indications that this is extremely effective in combating anxiety. However, start out carefully and build up slowly if you have suffered panic attacks or serious bouts of worry in the past; otherwise, you could bring on an anxious reaction if you start out too gung-ho.

If for some reason you can't or won't raise your heart rate, just go for a walk. This also has an anxiety-suppressing effect, though not quite as strong as if you were to move more briskly.

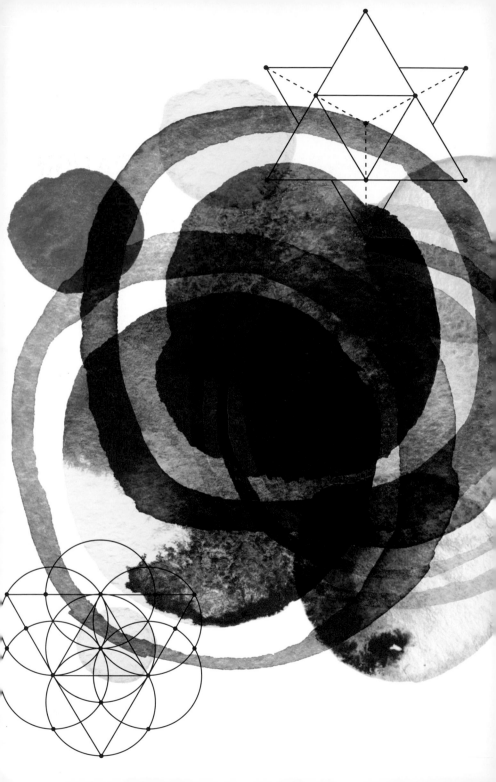

3. IMPROVED CONCENTRATION

Strength of mind is exercise, not rest.
ALEXANDER POPE

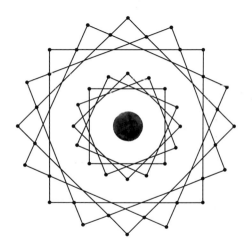

Do you sometimes find it hard to concentrate? If so, welcome to the club to which almost all of us belong. In today's world of information overload, where cell phones and computers jostle for our attention, it's virtually impossible to not get distracted. Being engrossed by a task and captivated by it to the point where time stands still is so rare—for me at least—that I almost consider it a luxury.

Fixing our flagging attention has become big business. There is a steady stream of self-help books, food supplements, and home remedies that are supposed to improve our powers of concentration, most of them having no proven merit whatsoever.

In truth, there is a remedy that not only helps but also makes a big difference; it is, once again, physical activity. It is only over the past few years that we've become able to show that we become more focused— and otherwise more alert—through exercise, as well as knowledgeable about what takes place inside the brain.

FOCUS ON ONE THING

Let's go back and start from the beginning. To see if anything can boost our powers of concentration, we must be able to measure this power. But how can it be done? Is it enough to simply ask someone if they're feeling focused? In science, you would want to have a more objective measure. Enter the Eriksen Flanker test, which consists of an exercise using five arrows on a monitor. The task is to indicate which direction the middle arrow points to, as quickly as possible. Occasionally all the arrows go in the same direction (<<<<<), which makes things easy. But sometimes the middle arrow points in one direction and the others go in the other direction (>><>>), so the trick is to ignore all the arrows except the middle one. The test is fast-paced; the arrows are only shown for two seconds. To quickly single out and focus on only part of what you see and ignore the rest of the information—in this case, the surrounding arrows—the brain needs to block out irrelevant information. This is called *selective attention.*

This type of test might seem pretty ordinary, but it is in fact an accurate indication of our ability to zero in on one thing and not become distracted by our surroundings. Selective attention is an important part of our ability to concentrate and a valuable trait in today's world. Imagine a day at the office: You're on the computer while two of your colleagues are chatting away, and someone else is running the printer. The phone pings at incoming texts and emails. You're trying to get your work done amid all of this, so it's important that you concentrate and not be sidetracked by all the buzz around you. This is selective attention, which is what the Eriksen Flanker test aims to measure.

The notion that exercise could affect selective attention and concentration became obvious when a group of people were given the Eriksen Flanker test. The participants' physical fitness levels were tested at the same time. It indicated that the participants who were fit did better on the test (i.e., they had better selective attention). But it doesn't end there. The test subjects' brains were also examined by MRI during the test, and it was noted that areas of the parietal lobe (in the middle of the skull) and the frontal lobe—parts of the brain that are vital to our ability to be and remain focused—were more active in the subjects who were in good shape. Activity in the areas important for concentration was higher in that sample of testers.

Be that as it may, we can't make too much of this information since we cannot say for sure that better selective attention is due to people's fitness. It could be the case that people who can concentrate harder tend to enjoy exercise and are therefore fitter, rather than the other way around. Consequently, the next step was to look at new test subjects, who were training to increase their fitness, to see if this would improve their selective attention. The participants were split into two groups: one group met three times a week to walk on a treadmill for forty-five minutes; the other group performed low-impact stretching exercises. They did this as many times and for the same duration as the walking group, with one key difference: they did not raise their heart rate.

Six months later, it was time to see if either group had improved at the Eriksen Flanker test and to check for any noticeable differences in the subjects' brains. And sure enough, there were differences! The walkers had not only improved their selective attention and did better on the test, but the activity in the areas of the frontal and parietal lobes responsible for selective attention ability showed changes, too. This effect was only seen in the participants who walked. Engaging in physical activity as simple and uncomplicated as regular walking for six months didn't simply improve selective attention; it produced a measurable effect on the brain.

Why is this the case? One possible explanation is that walking might have increased the amount of connections between brain cells in the frontal lobe, which made it easier for the brain to recruit additional mental capacity in these areas when the intellectual load became high. Like a car shifting into a higher gear, the brain makes use of an extra "focus gear" to stay on track when there are a lot of distractions around. We become more adept at filtering out what is unimportant. The study's authors could not have been any clearer when they stated that the end results showed "a brain that is more efficient, has better plasticity, and better adaptive capacity."

But how does training achieve this effect, and how can you exercise to improve your concentration? In this instance, the test subjects walked; but is running, biking, or swimming better? And for how long? The answers can be found in research that shows how physical training affects a specific condition, one in which the ability to concentrate is the issue itself. It's a diagnosis that has mushroomed over the past few years; we all see traces of it in ourselves to a lesser or greater degree: *Attention-deficit/hyperactivity disorder* (ADHD).

The ADHD epidemic

A Google search for the four letters *ADHD*, the acronym for attention-deficit/hyperactivity disorder, brings up fifty-three million results. ADHD has become our era's most recognized and discussed medical problem. It is also the diagnosis that has risen the most, by a wide margin. *Time* magazine warned around the turn of the millennium that too many children were being prescribed medication for ADHD and put the controversial question "Do we drug our children?" out there. At the time, between 4 and 5 percent of all American children and adolescents had been diagnosed with ADHD. Now, fifteen years later, these numbers look tame. We now estimate that 12 percent of the country's children and teenagers—over six million kids—have been diagnosed with ADHD.

This increase has been so explosive that, for a period, it was hard to find ADHD medication in the United States. The demand was so huge that pharmaceutical companies couldn't keep their production levels up.

We're all somewhere along the ADHD spectrum

A diagnosis of ADHD is built on the presumption that you have issues in three areas: concentration, impulsivity, and hyperactivity. Like the boy in class who could never sit still, who bounced around like a pinball, and who paid attention to everything except for what the teacher was writing on the blackboard. He acted on every little whim. There's no doubt that he had trouble concentrating and that he was impulsive and hyperactive—he ticked the three boxes for an ADHD diagnosis.

But do we have to be like him to suffer from ADHD? We all have difficulty focusing from time to time, but that doesn't mean that we all have ADHD. Concentration is affected by different elements, such as sleep, stress, the time of day, and what's in our environment. Furthermore, concentration can vary over long periods of time; the same goes for impulsivity and hyperactivity. So, where do we draw the line between what are run-of-the-mill concentration problems and what is ADHD? To put it mildly, that's not easy to figure out.

There are no blood tests or x-rays to tell you if you have ADHD. Instead, you must meet the conditions on a checklist of criteria. Other than having trouble with concentration, impulse control, and hyperactivity, these problems must also affect everyday living. Having problems at school is not enough, since that could be due to a poor academic environment. The problems should be apparent at home, at school, or in the workplace. The difficulties should also be obvious as early as childhood. ADHD isn't something you catch; it's a lifelong issue.

Being diagnosed with ADHD requires that you have serious problems with concentration and impulse control. What does this mean, exactly? If you've had issues with concentration but were still able to graduate from university, does that indicate that you don't have ADHD? At the risk of repeating myself here, there is no single answer to these questions. ADHD is, unlike many other medical diagnoses, a vast gray area. Without making any comparisons between ADHD and HIV other than the fact that they are both medical diagnoses, it's impossible to "have a little bit of HIV"—either you're infected, or you're not—but you can suffer from "a little bit of ADHD." An ADHD diagnosis is neither black nor white; it deals in qualities that are typically variable among us humans beings, and there is no clear line between ADHD and non-ADHD. We're all somewhere along the ADHD spectrum, and we exhibit characteristics for the diagnosis to a lesser or greater degree. Some of us have more of them than others.

THE REWARD SYSTEM IS THE BRAIN'S ENGINE

Keeping in mind that ADHD includes problems that many of us grapple with, it's wise to wonder if there's anything, aside from medication, that could be of help even for people with concentration problems that aren't sufficient to be diagnosed as ADHD. This is where exercise and training enter the picture. The connection between physical activity and concentration begins in an unexpected place, namely, in the area that makes you feel good when you eat tasty food, socialize with friends, or get praise at work: your brain's reward system.

The reward system is incredibly powerful and can be compared to an engine that pulls us toward certain behaviors. There are several important areas connected with reward, but the one we typically refer to when we say "reward center" is the *nucleus accumbens*—a pea-sized cluster of brain cells connected to many areas throughout the brain. This is where you get your "reward," your feeling of pleasure. The nucleus accumbens is what

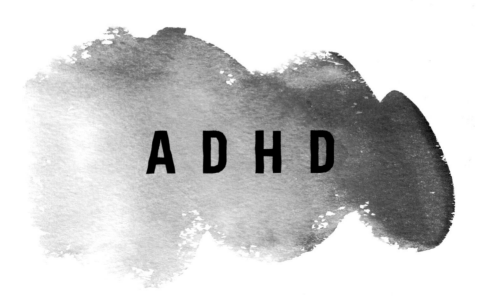

drives you. There are several substances that act as messengers between brain cells, and in scientific parlance they are known as *neurotransmitters*, of which dopamine is the best known. Certain behaviors, such as eating good food, socializing with others, being physically active, and having sex increase levels of dopamine in the nucleus accumbens. The spike of dopamine gives you a positive feeling, which makes you want to repeat those behaviors because your brain is pushing you to engage in them. Why does your brain want you to eat, socialize, be physically active, and have sex? The answer is simple: from an evolutionary perspective, these behaviors increase your chances of survival and ensure that you'll transmit your genes to the next generation. If there is a purely biological drive in life, it is to survive and transmit your genes (i.e., to have children), and the brain is programmed with that as its North Star. You need food to survive. Socializing with others is crucial for the survival of a herd animal, like a human. Having sex increases the likelihood of transmitting genes through procreation.

What about exercise; why does that make you feel good? Probably because when our ancestors ran, they usually did it as part of hunting or finding new places to settle—activities that promoted survival, which consequently were rewarded by the brain. Unlike us, our ancestors didn't run for the fun of it or for weight control, but because it increased their chances for survival. That's why we also benefit from being physically active, even today.

No concentration without reward

By rewarding behaviors with good feelings, the nucleus accumbens steers you toward whatever actions increase your chances of survival and the transmittal of your genes. But the reward system is not only there to make you feel warm and fuzzy; it is also central to your ability to concentrate. The nucleus accumbens isn't off most the time and turned on only because you're eating a good meal, having sex, or finding out that you've won the lottery. It's always active and providing feedback to the rest of your brain

Our ancestors ran not because it was enjoyable or to control their weight, but because it increased their chances of survival. That's why we also benefit from being physically active.

about whether what you're up to is worth continuing or not. Let's say you're watching television. If your nucleus accumbens isn't stimulated enough by the program (i.e., if your dopamine levels aren't elevated), your attention will shift and you'll look elsewhere for a hit of dopamine—maybe from what's on your cell phone. If you constantly lose focus and scan your surroundings for something interesting, you'll be perceived as restless and distracted.

Today we know that the reward system appears to be different from person to person. In some, it's finely tuned as soon as they're born, while in others it works less well. Many things indicate that people with significant concentration issues have a reward system that runs differently. What increases the dopamine levels for most of us isn't enough for them.

Their reward system requires more stimuli to become active, and that has major consequences. A reward system that is always underactivated will lead people to constantly change their focus and hunt for something that will give them a larger thrill. They opt for what delivers the best, most immediate pleasurable experience and ignore what is good for them in the long run. They have trouble setting up and following long-term goals and are interrupted by distractions big and small. They become careless, impulsive, and, in some cases, hyperactive.

Many who have trouble focusing do learn a variety of strategies to cope with this, such as organizing their life and having clear routines to follow throughout the day. When things become turbulent, those routines are a buffer from distraction.

It has been shown that the nucleus accumbens isn't as active when a person with great concentration problems—someone with ADHD, for instance—is exposed to what normally would be considered a reward. More stimuli seem to be required to activate his or her reward center.

Too few receivers in the reward center

Nowadays we've begun to understand, at the molecular level, why there are differences in the reward centers of different people. For dopamine to have an effect in the reward center and to make you feel good, it must be able to bind to a receptor on the surface of the brain cell. The dopamine plugs in to the receptor, which sets off a reaction in the brain cell that makes you feel pleasure. However, nothing happens if there is no receptor for the dopamine to plug into, and the reaction does not occur. Interestingly, it looks like people with ADHD have fewer dopamine receptors in their reward centers. This means that their reward systems don't work well, and that they require greater rewards to be responsive.

This means that there are some people whose brain, from the onset, demands more stimulation to activate the reward center. What someone with a normal reward center deems sufficiently interesting to keep his or her attention—a work task, a television series, or what the teacher is writing on the blackboard—is not adequate; it doesn't create enough activity in the reward center. This person becomes bored and attempts, subconsciously, to find further stimulation in some other way, and consequently loses his or her concentration. Concentrating on work or on what the teacher is writing becomes impossible. Then again, all of us are perched somewhere along the ADHD spectrum. We don't have a reward system that works normally, yet we don't have one that totally malfunctions. Most of us find ourselves somewhere in the middle.

68

WORLD CHAMPION OF BAD DECISIONS

"If there were such a thing, I would probably have been crowned world champion of bad decision making. I have always chosen what works for me in the present moment, damn the long-term consequences. I could never sit still in school and had to be in a special education class where everyone behaved much like I did. My grades were awful, and I ended up running with a bad crowd and experimenting with drugs by the time I was thirteen. I quite quickly discovered amphetamines, which became my drug of choice. What made other people hyper had a calming effect on me.

"Naturally, the combination of drugs and risk taking was a recipe for disaster, and as my drug addiction become more expensive, my criminal activities turned serious. It all ended with a spell in prison.

"When I told my story to the prison doctor, he diagnosed me with ADHD. After I was put on medication I could suddenly focus—my life got clearer, and I began to get things done. It became easier to function every day and to socialize with friends; I could be present and not feel perpetually out of it, as if I were somewhere else."

This forty-four-year-old man's story is pretty typical; I've heard similar accounts from hundreds of other patients. While each one of them suffered great strife due to a lack of concentration and impulse control, not many of them became addicts or criminals. What is striking is that this man looks markedly well trained and is very fit. He had made working out a priority his entire life despite his otherwise self-destructive ways, because he would feel calm after exhausting himself physically: "[After working out] I'd be like everyone else and could listen to others without being distracted by everything around me. Now I realize that, throughout my life, working out has been a type of ADHD medication."

Consciousness and attention

The greatest mystery of the brain, and perhaps of all scientific mysteries, is how this collection of cells inside the cranium, weighing only slightly more than a kilogram (2¼ lbs), becomes conscious. How it turns into *you*. It was long believed that it was frivolous for scientists to even *attempt* to understand consciousness, a bit like trying to search for the meaning of life. But today's scientific research into the conscious mind is as far from silly as you can get. Recent medical discoveries have provided us with a whole new set of tools for studying consciousness. It's not only a matter of interest to neuroscientists; physicists, psychologists, and philosophers are also trying their best to figure out the riddle of how some cells—because that's what we're made of, after all—can become aware of their own existence. How can they even comprehend how they are built and what place they occupy in the universe's space and time continuum?

Where did this research lead us to? Where is our consciousness located? The short answer is: we don't know. We don't even know what consciousness is. Some of history's great thinkers have put forth some ideas. Plato, for instance, didn't believe our mortal body could create a consciousness. Polymath Leonardo da Vinci leaned toward the theory that consciousness was most likely connected to the brain but located in its fluid-filled cavities (i.e., the cerebral ventricles). The philosopher René Descartes suggested that our consciousness was situated in the pineal gland, a small gland in the brain that we now know secretes the hormone melatonin, which regulates sleep and wakefulness.

No disrespect intended, but modern neurological research has proven the aforementioned geniuses to be mistaken. Today, no one disputes the fact that our consciousness is *in fact* in the brain, and that it is not in one singular location. Our senses of smell, sight, and hearing all have specific centers, but there isn't a lone consciousness center. Instead, it seems that many areas in the cerebral cortex make up and work as an advanced network, and that consciousness is the result of the collaboration between the frontal and the temporal lobe, along with the centers for sensory impressions (like the sight and hearing centers).

The *thalamus* is the part of the brain that acts like a junction. It is situated in the brain like the hub on a bicycle's wheel, from which the spokes extend outward. To illustrate: information is brought into the thalamus from the brain's different areas, like the centers for sensory impressions, and from there the data are spread out to the other areas through the advanced network. It is within this network that we believe our experience of consciousness is created.

What does all this have to do with concentration? Well, consciousness isn't just fascinating from a philosophical and scientific point of view; it is also closely connected to our ability to pay attention and focus. Your brain is constantly filled to bursting with activity, where information from different areas compete for a spot in your consciousness. You're fed sensory information about what position your legs and arms are currently in, if the room is warm or cold, if you're feeling pain anywhere, and what you're seeing and hearing right now—which could be the words in this sentence or a car sounding its horn out in the street. Your consciousness sifts through all of this and decides what your brain should concentrate on—hopefully, it's this sentence!—and what is unimportant.

Dopamine turns off the din

Let's say you're in a coffee shop and you're reading a book. First, you're aware of the murmur of the people in the background, but that sound slowly recedes and you can concentrate on what you're reading. Even though you're no longer listening to the voices, your brain still registers what is being said. If someone in the coffee shop says your name, you'll probably react even though you weren't actively listening. Part of your brain must still be hearing, without you being aware of it, and you'll turn your attention in that direction. Obviously, this happens automatically. The brain possesses the amazing ability to process huge numbers of impressions without us being in on it, sounding the alarm and focusing our attention on what is deemed important.

We need dopamine to turn down the din that our sensory centers bombard us with and to direct our attention toward whatever we are doing. Dopamine has considerably more responsibilities than just being a rewards compound; it is also critical for concentration. Lacking dopamine can lead us to become unfocused and jittery, distracted by background noise. We all go through this sometimes; we'll feel unsettled, jumpy, and absentminded, especially if we've slept badly or we've drunk alcohol the night before.

Oddly enough, there's another kind of din in your head, a kind of inbuilt hum that doesn't originate in the sensory centers. It's something we all experience, and it doesn't mean we're going crazy. It's probably caused by brain cells activating spontaneously from time to time. This happens continuously, but you probably don't notice it because dopamine filters it out. However, without a finely tuned dopamine system, that interior noise—like the din from sensory centers—can become bothersome. Neurological tests have shown that persons with ADHD have a louder inbuilt hum that disturbs and impairs their ability to concentrate. The more interior noise there is, the worse the focus.

It's interesting to note that if dopamine levels increase, the interior, non-stimulus-driven thrum will stop. Both the noise from your sensory centers (the din in the café, for example) and the inbuilt hum call it quits. It's like hearing the irritating sound of static in the background because no station is tuned in—and the dopamine lowers the volume and silences the hiss. There's no more disturbance, and it gets easier to focus.

NATURAL CONCENTRATION MEDICATION

Low or incorrectly regulated dopamine levels can cause a din, which keeps the dopamine system insufficiently activated and makes it difficult to concentrate. Therefore, the obvious next step would be to try

72

and treat the lack of focus, and increase and stabilize dopamine levels through artificial means. That's the mechanism behind most ADHD medications: they boost dopamine levels, which in turn lead to improved focus. Many ADHD sufferers claim that their existence becomes sharper and clearer, which probably stems from the fact that the hum in their brain—internal and external—has been silenced. However, not everyone who's on medication experiences this. Also, not everyone wants to take medication. Add to this all the people who occasionally have trouble concentrating without suffering from full-blown ADHD. Is there any other way to boost dopamine levels without resorting to pharmaceuticals? There is: move your body.

Possibly the most important reason why exercise is good for concentration—whether you suffer from ADHD or not—is that physical activity raises dopamine levels and fine-tunes the systems for attention and reward. Today, we know that dopamine levels increase at first *after* you've been physically active. They rise a few minutes after a training session, and they remain there for several hours. This makes you feel sharp, focused, and calm after exercising. You feel better, and it's easier for you to concentrate. The hum is hushed.

It appears that the more strenuous the exercise, the higher dopamine levels rise, so from dopamine's standpoint, going for a run is better than going for a walk. It's all the more reason why you shouldn't give up after your first run or bike ride if you don't feel better right away or if your focus has not improved. The more you train, the more dopamine you'll get. The brain seems to increase it more and more, so the more often you run on the trail or cycle that loop, the greater your dopamine reward. This means you'll feel better every time you complete a session, since dopamine also affects your feeling of well-being, and your concentration will improve even more. In other words, exercise is effective medicine for improving concentration, with no side effects whatsoever. Furthermore, its effect is enhanced the longer you continue.

Brain boss

Dopamine has many important effects on the frontal lobe (which is located directly behind your frontal bone). It's the frontal lobe, especially its anterior part—the prefrontal cortex—that makes the decisions in the brain. The prefrontal cortex is the brain's boss, and its most developed area. The ability to set and follow through on long-term goals, instead of simply acting on impulse, is found here. The same is true for our advanced cognitive functions—those that separate us from other animals—such as abstract, mathematical, and logical thinking.

It is also the frontal lobe that is largely responsible for controlling our ability to concentrate. Simply put, we have a lot of turbulence in the deeper reaches of the brain. The frontal lobe suppresses this commotion and behaves like a filter that removes the noise and allows us to focus.

The ability to wait for reward

How the frontal lobe works plays a pivotal role in the way our lives turn out. In the 1970s, professor of psychology Walter Mischel revealed that children's ability to delay a reward—a function that exists primarily in the frontal lobe—can predict their future personality profile. Mischel's test in delayed gratification showed four-year-old children who had to choose between enjoying a marshmallow right away or two marshmallows if they could wait twenty minutes to get them. Most of the kids found the temptation too great and could only wait two to three minutes before eating the treat. Some children could restrain themselves a little longer, and some managed to hold out for the entire twenty minutes in order to get the two marshmallows.

Mischel followed these test subjects for several decades and noted that those who could delay gratification did, on average, better academically, reaching higher educational levels as adults. They've encountered fewer problems with alcohol abuse, drugs, and obesity. They also handle stress better. The variances in how people's frontal lobes function are visible early in life and have lifelong consequences.

Exercise is effective medicine for improving concentration, with no side effects whatsoever.

To control the impulse to eat the candy requires a great deal of discipline from a four-year-old child (this is true for adults, too), which is a function that is connected to concentration. An important reason why some children do better on the test than others is that they are able to focus better, thus succeeding in zeroing in on the future reward. In a video of the study, you can see some children straining to the breaking point, kicking frantically against the chair in front of them to distract themselves. When those who could wait were asked how they did it, many replied that they thought intensely about the fact that they would soon get two marshmallows.

This kind of concentration and ability to delay gratification are executive functions also known as *cognitive control*, which are part of what Walter Mischel calls the brain's "cooling system." The Nobel Prize winner Daniel Kahneman calls it "System 2"—the brain's slower, more deliberate system. Other scientists and authors throughout history have used different designations, but they all basically refer to the same thing: the system we have for our higher thinking that keeps a lid on impulses and has its origin in the frontal lobe and prefrontal cortex. It's a system that is strengthened in many ways when we are physically active.

You control your brain, not the other way around
As you saw earlier in the chapter *Run away from stress*, the frontal lobe is one of the brain's areas that is strengthened the most by physical exercise.

The frontal lobe of a person who works out regularly becomes better connected to other parts of the brain, which is critical for its ability to influence and control the rest of the brain. New blood vessels are also created in the frontal lobes in people who are physically active, which allows for better blood supply and removal of waste products. The processes that lead your walks or runs to a stronger frontal lobe are powerful, but not immediate. You won't notice anything different after one loop around the track, but rather after several months of regular activity.

Because the frontal lobe is changeable and malleable, the marshmallow test's creator, Walter Mischel, is careful to stress that the test does not mean that those who can't resist temptations are condemned to have problems later in life. You can practice resisting temptations, and physical activity is probably a very important step in doing this. It is not your brain that controls you—it is you who control your brain through your actions. If you want to ensure the best possible conditions for yourself, stay physically active.

CHILDREN WITH ADHD NEED EXERCISE AND PLAY

When you come to terms with how important the frontal lobe and dopamine are for concentration—and how they are influenced by exercise—you realize that, at least in theory, it should be possible to treat ADHD with physical training. But as you know, theory and practice don't always converge, so what does the research tell us? Is exercise so effective in sharpening our concentration that we can even use it to treat ADHD?

A group of scientists decided to explore this question by using seventeen children as test subjects, all of whom exhibited such hyperactive behavior that they were at risk of being diagnosed with ADHD. Over the course of eight weeks, the kids enjoyed extra physical activity in the form of play before the start of the school day. The goal was to get them winded and raise their heart rate. At the end of those eight weeks, the kids performed a battery of tests that measured their ability

76

> *It's not your brain that rules you—it is you who rule your brain through your actions.*

to concentrate and socialize with other children. Additionally, the kids' parents and teachers were asked if they had noticed any progress.

Did all this activity have any effect? It did. According to the parents, teachers, researchers, and instructors, more than two-thirds of the children were reported to be more focused. Progress was noted especially in what is called *response-inhibition*, the ability to suppress actions and to not act impulsively on every little thing, which tends to be very difficult for children with ADHD.

Despite those promising results, it couldn't be ignored that this was only a very small study, so the same test was repeated on over two hundred children. It was estimated that half of the test subjects were at high risk of being labeled ADHD. Over the course of twelve weeks, the children played in groups for half an hour each day, with the goal of getting their heart rates up. As a control group, one set of children engaged in quieter activities, such as painting and drawing.

The scientists decided to forgo the battery of psychological tests and simply asked parents and teachers, who were in daily contact with the children, how they perceived them. They were asked to judge how the children had changed in terms of attention span, hyperactivity, ability to focus, and how they got along with other kids. The children in the group who got to play didn't merely improve their ability to focus; they also experienced fewer mood swings and threw fewer temper tantrums. A real difference was felt at home. And while this effect was noted in all the children who had been allowed to play, hyper or not, the biggest impact was seen in the kids who were thought to have ADHD.

This is more than simply burning off excess energy

The test subjects participated in regular physical activity over several months, but positive effects on concentration are swift to manifest themselves—as little as a single five-minute exercise session improves concentration and lessens ADHD symptoms in children! Perhaps you think they simply burned off some excess energy, which was why they calmed down. It wasn't quite as simple as that. The impact on their concentration was far too significant to be simply due to exhaustion.

Everyone's concentration improves

So far, the tests I've described have focused on how physical activity affects concentration in people with ADHD, primarily in children. But what about us, adults who do not have ADHD? Can we, too, expect to see an effect on our powers of concentration? Absolutely! Vivid proof of this can be found in the outcome of a test performed on two hundred pairs of seventeen-year-old identical twins. To measure the twins' day-to-day levels of concentration, scientists decided to let their parents grade the twins in fourteen different categories, including attention, hyperactivity, and impulsivity. Three years later, when the twins were in their twenties, the parents conducted another round of grading, which showed that most of the twins had gained better concentration over that span of time. However, one group stood out by having markedly improved their ability to focus, and it was the twins who had been physically active in their free time. The more intensely physical the activity, the more concentration improved.

This was evident even within a pair of twins, in which one twin was active and the other was not. In those cases, the twin who exercised had better concentration than his or her sibling. The results were due to differences in lifestyle, not on genes or environment. The interesting fact here is that this study analyzed people in their twenties who did not have ADHD; nevertheless, it was obvious that the twins who were physically active showed better concentration and impulse control than the

As short as a five-minute training session improves concentration and lessens symptoms of ADHD.

sedentary twins. The improvement wasn't immediate but happened over time; there was a three-year gap between the parents' ratings, after all.

WHY IS CONCENTRATION IMPROVED BY MOVEMENT?

Indeed, why is concentration improved by movement? We can answer that by looking to the past, because it's probably thanks to our ancestors and their lives on the savanna. They were physically active for reasons other than those that drive you and me to run on a treadmill. Today, most of us run because it makes us feel good, it's healthy for us, and it keeps our weight under control. Our forefathers probably didn't think about that stuff. They ran to catch food or to avoid danger; in either case, you'd better pay attention. There's no room for error when there's a lion behind you or when you're getting ready to catch an antelope. Sharpened concentration is a survival asset in such situations. Your chances for survival increase with your brain's ability to harness additional focus. Our brains haven't evolved much more since our ancestors' days on the savanna, so it's the same mechanism that comes into play today, even when we exercise: the brain believes that we're engaging potentially vital activity that requires an all-out effort, which leads us to concentrate better.

ADHD can also be an advantage

We often consider attention disorders and ADHD to be negative attributes. That's not surprising, since symptoms must become a problem before a diagnosis can be made. However, qualities such as impulsivity

79

and hyperactivity can also be turned to our advantage. Many restless and driven people get things accomplished because they don't have the patience to wait around for results. It's no accident that many successful business leaders and entrepreneurs have personality traits that call to mind the characteristics of ADHD.

The Ariaal tribe from the desert of northern Kenya is a good illustration of how ADHD need not be a negative trait. The tribe's members live the same way today as they did thousands of years ago, constantly moving livestock in their search for water and food. However, in the past few decades the tribe has split into groups. One group has put down stakes in one location and lives off agriculture, while the other has kept up its nomadic, hunter-gatherer lifestyle.

Scientists examined the tribe members' genetic profile through blood tests—what interested them specifically was a gene that's essential for dopamine in the brain. The gene, called DRD_4, is present in all human beings, and it plays an important role in concentration. DRD_4 has a few variations, one of which is more common in people with ADHD. Although no single gene can cause ADHD, and even DRD_4 by itself can't be held responsible for it, it is one of the single most important genes involved in ADHD.

The tests revealed that certain tribe members carried the DRD_4 variant connected to ADHD (it's a bit clunky, but I'll call it the *ADHD-variation of the gene* for now). Other members carried the regular variation of the gene—the gene not linked to ADHD. This was not unexpected. What was a surprise, however, was that the nomads of the tribe who carried the ADHD-variation of the gene were better nourished than those who expressed the regular variation of the gene. In other words, hunter-gatherers carrying the ADHD-variation of the gene seemed to have an easier time finding food than the hunters without the ADHD gene. The situation was reversed when the farmers were examined. The ADHD-gene carriers were undernourished compared to those who didn't carry the gene. It appears the ADHD gene is an advantage to the hunters, but a drawback for the farmers, which illustrates that the same gene can be a plus for people living in one type of environment and a weakness for people living in another. But we can't blame outcomes on people's different genetic origins, because the Ariaal tribe only split into farmers and hunter-gatherers a few decades ago. Instead, one conclusion we can draw from these observations is that the qualities we link to ADHD—namely, impulsivity and hyperactivity—can be an advantage for hunters in an energetic environment in which they need to make quick decisions. On the other hand, the need for farmers to act quickly isn't as urgent, since it's more important, in their environment, to concentrate on long-term results and work patiently, a situation in which ADHD traits might be a hindrance.

The perfect ADHD environment

That the ADHD gene seems to be useful for the Ariaal tribe's hunters points to something interesting. There is reason to believe that even among our hunting ancestors (which most of them were until about ten thousand years ago, at which time agriculture developed), there was a benefit to carrying this type of genetic heritage. In an environment where you hike, hunt, and move from place to place depending on where the food is, restlessness and impulsivity may mean that you have energy to make snap decisions. It's almost perfect for someone who has ADHD. We've lived in that kind of environment for most of humanity's history. From that perspective, we realize that the traits we associate today with ADHD have, historically speaking, been a boon. Conversely, if impulsivity and hyperactivity had caused only problems and had not provided some advantages, we would hardly encounter so many people with ADHD nowadays, since these characteristics would have been wiped out by natural selection.

Interestingly, the ADHD gene isn't an advantage for just hunters; it also seems to be more common in nomadic populations (I don't mean "nomadic" in the way we change apartments or jobs every so often;

I use the term to refer to primitive people who move around frequently). The gene appears to be associated with the desire to move around and explore new environments—a sort of "explorer gene," if you will.

The human race originated in East Africa and gradually made its way across the planet over the past one hundred thousand years. Discovering new environments and seeking out unknown vistas is a fundamental trait in our nature and has been crucial to our survival. We can suppose that this underlying drive to explore comes, to a great extent, from individuals who exhibit personality traits that we would now associate with ADHD.

The brain is built for movement

The Ariaal tribe isn't the only case in which one lone gene can have both advantages and disadvantages depending on the environment in which it is expressed. It's the same in our society, too. Characteristics that cause trouble in one social context or in one type of workplace might seem favorable in another. The problem is that there are no longer many occasions in which ADHD qualities are an asset. Risk taking and impulsivity are rarely viewed with approval in today's world. These are types of behaviors we try to avoid and actively discourage in our children.

In other words, that ADHD may have an advantage if you are a hunter on the savanna is a moot point. We don't hunt for our food; we buy it at the grocery store. Having a gene that predisposes us to explore new environments isn't that great a deal, either. We won't be rewarded for finding a new, unknown fertile valley where we can settle down, because there aren't any to be found. Instead, we'll be punished for not being able to sit still. The sensory hypersensitivity that is inherent to many with ADHD means they'd be able to see the tiniest movements of their prey on the savanna, which in turn would increase the likelihood of their catching it. However, in school students are punished when the smallest sound distracts them and renders them unable to concentrate on what the teacher is writing on the blackboard. Ours is a challenging time to live in for someone with ADHD. What was considered helpful at one time has become a bane to our modern, urban society—and something that we try to medicate away.

From an evolutionary standpoint, looking at ADHD as only a problem is too obtuse. We also know that there are other ways besides pharmaceuticals to try to solve issues that arise from ADHD. One way is to change your lifestyle and try to live the way we have evolved to. We can't go back to the savanna, but we can go running on a trail or hit the gym. If we do, we'll be better equipped to handle the world we have changed so quickly, one that puts such high demands on our cognitive abilities.

Maybe that's why training has such good results on people who have ADHD. They meet the physical challenges that we encountered so naturally in our distant past, which seems so vital to them. Everyone has a brain that is built for movement, but the brain of someone with ADHD is especially attuned to movement! Just as exercise and physical training help the ADHD sufferer to focus, it can assist the rest of us whose attention occasionally goes on a walkabout. After all, we're all perched somewhere along the ADHD spectrum.

As you've seen in this chapter, having trouble concentrating isn't due to just one thing. The nucleus accumbens (i.e., the reward center) might be calibrated differently in different people, which affects concentration. The brain's interior din levels can vary, and the frontal lobe might be more, or less, competent at quieting the noise and honing our attention.

In other words, there can be a multitude of reasons for why our concentration is flagging; what all of them seem to have in common is that they are affected by our level of physical activity. Furthermore, once we change our sedentary habits for the better, our ability to concentrate improves.

Counteract the din with exercise

Today, we produce as much digital information over two days as we've done in the entire history of humanity up to the year 2003. We are drowning in the data generated from our computers and smartphones, a stream that doesn't appear to be slowing down anytime soon. Meanwhile, our brain, which we expect to handle this incredible overload of information, has hardly changed at all the in past several thousands of years.

It isn't particularly surprising that our concentration wanes occasionally and that we need all the help we can get to accommodate this flow of information. The knee-jerk response to this issue cannot just consist of more diagnoses and more prescription medication. We should also look at our lifestyle and see what changes we can make to improve our concentration.

Research clearly indicates that what truly puts our extra "mental concentration" gear to work is physical exercise, not diet supplements or apps with cognitive exercises. Physical activity makes us better equipped to meet a world that looks less and less like the one we evolved for. It's in this light that you should look at training and its effects on concentration. I hope that this chapter has helped you realize—whether you're suffering from ADHD or not, whether you're a kid or an adult—what good movement can do for your ability to focus.

TOO MUCH COUCH-SURFING IS DETRIMENTAL TO YOUR THINKING

You have probably seen the headlines about how spending a lot of time sitting can increase your risk of acquiring a whole host of illnesses. In fact, physical inactivity has even worse consequences: you'll think more slowly and poorly. American scientists followed just over 3,200 young Americans for twenty-five years, during which time information was recorded about how physically active they were and how much time they spent in front of the television. In addition, different psychological tests were performed to gauge their memory, concentration skills, and cognitive processing speed (i.e., how quickly they could think).

The tests clearly indicated that the test subjects who were sedentary had inferior powers of concentration and memory. They also thought more slowly. The difference was huge. The results from subjects who sat for long periods of time and watched TV for at least three hours a day were especially lousy. The expression "boob tube" is indeed very meaningful!

Much of this book is about the immediate effects exercise has on your brain, but in this case the results were very gradual, since the individuals were followed over a period of twenty-five years. It shows how important physical activity is for our mental abilities, even over the long haul. Being sedentary too much not only makes you unfocused, anxious, and depressed; it also makes you think slower because it impairs your cognitive skills.

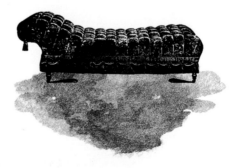

Exercise and physical training help ADHD sufferers to concentrate—and it works for the rest of us, too. We are, after all, all perched somewhere along the ADHD spectrum.

IMPROVED CONCENTRATION

THE RIGHT PRESCRIPTION FOR IMPROVED CONCENTRATION

Go for a run instead of taking a walk. If you move more strenuously, your brain will release more dopamine and noradrenaline. Ideally, your heart rate should reach 70 to 75 percent of its maximum capacity. If you're forty, that translates to a reading of 130 to 140 bpm. If you're fifty years old, your reading should be at least 125.

Exercise in the morning. To target concentration, it's better to work out early in the day, or at least before noon, to let the effects last through the remainder of the day. The effect will taper off after a few hours, and most of us need to focus during the day, not in the evening.

Train for thirty minutes if you can. You should be active for at least twenty minutes, but thirty minutes is better to enjoy the full benefits.

Keep up the workouts! It takes a while for the effects of exercise on concentration (as well as on stress and general well-being) to take place, so don't give up! You must be patient to reap these rewards.

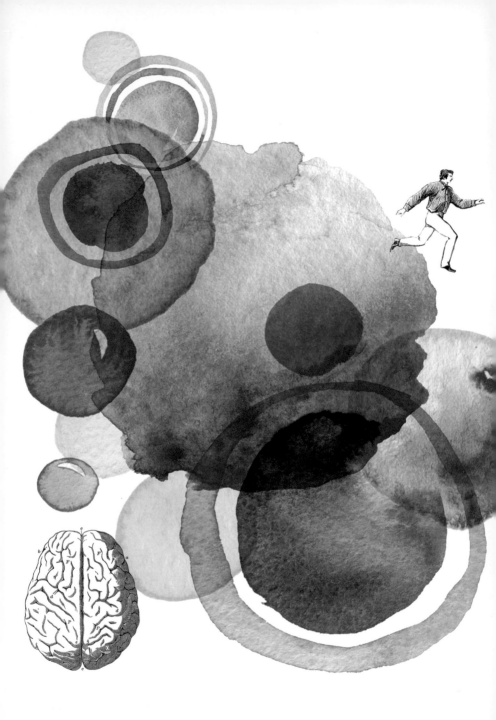

4. THE *REAL* HAPPY PILL

If you are in a bad mood, go for a walk.
If you are still in a bad mood, go for another walk.
HIPPOCRATES

One November evening a few years ago, a colleague at the hospital's emergency department where I worked asked me to see a woman in her forties. I was given a brief history, which only contained a few sentences: "Previously healthy woman. Extremely fatigued for the past twenty-four hours. Tests and CT (Computed Tomography)—also CAT—scan normal. Depression?"

The woman told me that she was feeling overwhelmingly tired that day. She was convinced that she had contracted some unusual disease and refused to believe that the results of all the tests recently performed on her had come back normal. "You must have missed something," she said. At first, she didn't understand what I was getting at when I asked what her life had been like recently, but then she explained that the past year had been very demanding. She was unhappy at work because her workload had not only increased, but her tasks had also become less and less clear. She and her husband had also bought a house, which they were in the process of renovating. That she had a lot on her plate, professionally and personally, was nothing new. This was the normal run of things for her, and it had never affected her before.

This fall, however, everything was different. She felt increasingly more exhausted. She became more and more withdrawn and didn't bother to keep up with friends. She used to enjoy horseback riding—she had ridden competitively—and reading, but she had not been to the stables in over a year and could hardly remember the last time she cracked open a book. The urge wasn't there anymore, and she couldn't focus long enough to read.

That morning when she woke up, she could hardly get out of bed. It was as if she had become paralyzed by her lethargy, and eventually her husband brought her to the emergency room. My colleague, who first saw her, thought it might be an infection, but the blood tests were clear. Even a CT scan of the patient's brain was completely normal and didn't reveal anything suspect. The woman hesitated when my colleague suggested that she meet with a psychiatrist. After all, what she was suffering from was physical! Besides, she had never had any mental problems in her life.

This woman suffered from depression, not from some obscure malady that the physicians had missed. Once she realized this, she asked me how it could be treated. I explained that she had to slow down her commitments a little bit, maybe even take some time off work or work fewer hours, and that we could give antidepression medication a try. There was also therapy. Her mother had taken antidepressants but they had undesirable side effects, so the patient didn't want to take any pills; she was also hesitant about therapy. Was there anything else she could do? I explained that exercise had the same impact on depression as medication, but it would require that she take up running for at least thirty minutes at a time, and preferably three times a week. It would take several weeks to take effect, but once it did, the outcome would be on par with that of antidepressants.

In her case, running three times a week was not a realistic goal, so we decided that she should start off with regular walks. She only managed ten-minute increments in the first few days, but gradually the walks got longer, and then faster. She was still tired when I met her at the hospital three weeks later, but she did have the energy to jog slowly, fifteen minutes at a time.

As the weeks went by, my patient upped her efforts. Four months after her initial visit to the ER, she was running three times a week, often close to an hour at a time. The transformation in her well-being was remarkable! She explained that she not only felt and slept better but also functioned better all around. Her short-term memory and concentration had improved. Her anxiety over trivialities was gone, and she didn't overreact as much to stress, whether work-related or at home. She had resumed horseback riding and reconnected with her friends. In addition, she had dealt with her situation at work and gotten clearer instructions on what was expected of her. According to her family, the difference was striking—"Mom is back."

What made her especially happy was that she *herself* had set in motion these changes by getting out there on the running trail. It took a Herculean effort at the beginning, but it became easier after a while. As this was due to her very own efforts, it did wonders for her self-esteem.

ONLY SICK AND EXHAUSTED, OR DEPRESSED?

Most of us will feel down and glum at one time or another. However, you are depressed if you are sad week after week, feel despondent when thinking about the future, and no longer find contentment in participating in the activities you typically enjoyed. How depression expresses itself varies from person to person: some feel so exhausted that they can hardly get out of bed in the morning, while others feel so anxious that they can't sleep at night. Some lose their appetite and weight falls off them, while others become hungry and quickly put on weight. There are many types of depression, but they all have as common denominator the enormous suffering they cause in those who are afflicted by it.

Today, almost everyone knows that you can treat depression with medication. Many are also aware that exercise is good for one's well-being, but most don't know just *how big* an impact it has, and that training is, in and of itself, an antidepressant. It is a medication without any

> *Training is, in and of itself, an antidepressant. It is medication without any side effects, which in most cases makes everyone feel better.*

side effects and that in most cases makes everyone feel better—whether you just feel a bit blue or you're in the grip of a deep depression.

Training works on all types of depressions

It's often challenging to properly define what constitutes depression; many of us can feel out of sorts for a while without being depressed. A list of nine criteria is used to diagnose depression: exhibiting a depressed or irritable mood; losing interest in things that used to be fun; inability to sleep well at night or sleeping too much; restlessness or an inability to sit still; fatigue and loss of energy; feeling worthless or guilty; having trouble concentrating; losing or gaining a lot of weight; and having recurring thoughts about death or suicide. At least five of those nine conditions should be met in order to diagnose depression. But what if you only check four of the criteria on the list? You may feel completely worthless, and everything seems futile. Your appetite is almost gone, and your sleep is lousy. It's obvious you're not feeling well, but it is not, clinically speaking, depression. This example illustrates the fact that psychiatry is not an exact science. Basically, these are all subjective experiences. Neither blood tests nor x-rays can tell if you're depressed or not. We use these checklists (which you can find online) in the psychiatric profession for lack of a better method, and they should be considered a means of help and not the absolute truth. Like ADHD, depression is a large gray zone.

If we prescribe an antidepressant to someone who is not suffering from depression, the medication typically has no effect. However, the effects of exercise are measurable, even for people who are simply down in the dumps and not miserable enough to be diagnosed with depression. Regardless of the level of depression, training makes everyone feel better, as the negative thoughts ebb away and self-esteem gets a boost.

Many of my patients are surprised when I tell them that running has the same effect as antidepressants, since few have heard of this. It's normal to wonder why so many don't know that regular runs can be just as effective as pharmaceuticals in the fight against depression. Most seem to harbor the belief that "if it were true, wouldn't everyone know about this already?" The reason for this widespread ignorance is very simple—it boils down to money.

PROZAC VERSUS TRAINING

On December 29, 1987, the powerful American government agency, the Food and Drug Administration (the FDA), decided to approve the sale of the medication Fluoxetine, making it the first new type of antidepressant available in the United States in almost two decades. This pharmaceutical became an enormous success even though it was introduced at a time when many still weren't convinced that depression had biological roots, or even that it originated in the brain. Fluoxetine was marketed under the name *Prozac*, and in short order it became not only one of the most widely sold drugs in the world, but also one of its best-known brands ever.

Thousands of articles and several books, among them the cult memoir *Prozac Nation*, were written about this new pill. The rapper Jay-Z sang about it, and even the character Tony Soprano, of TV's *The Sopranos* fame, was on Prozac.

Fluoxetine prevents brain cells from reabsorbing serotonin, thereby increasing the amount of active serotonin that is still available *between* the brain cells. Fluoxetine belongs to a group of pharmaceuticals called *selective serotonin reuptake inhibitors* (SSRIs). Within just a few years, several similar drugs were released in the marketplace, and they all became hugely successful and were taken by millions of people all over the world. But as sales skyrocketed, it became obvious that about one-third of the users saw no effects, and another third experienced only limited relief—even though they felt better, they were still depressed. Many users experienced side effects such as sleep disturbances, dry mouth, nausea, and low libido. Some of the side effects were only temporary, but they were still unpleasant enough that some people stopped taking the medication before it had time to become effective.

Doctors, scientists, and not least those who suffered from depression, began to wonder if there were other treatment options that didn't involve pharmaceuticals. It's not surprising that they chose to look into physical activity. As early as 1905, the psychiatric journal *The American Journal of Insanity*—a title that would not cut the mustard today—published a scientific article about the connection between exercise and how we feel.

At the end of 1980, we began to systematically compare the effect of training to that of medication on depression. The objective was to find out whether training could provide the same effects as pharmaceuticals.

Naturally, this research was not funded by pharmaceutical companies—businesses that would have had no commercial interest in seeing if training could cure depression—but by medical schools. This explains why the studies' budgets were a great deal smaller than the budgets provided by pharmacies when a new pharmaceutical is under development.

A breakthrough happened when American psychologist James Blumenthal gathered 156 individuals—a large group, given the field—who all suffered from depression. Blumenthal randomly assigned the subjects to three different groups. One group was given Zoloft, one of the most widely prescribed antidepressant drugs. Another group exercised for thirty minutes, three times a week. The last group both exercised and took the medication.

Four months later, it was time to check the results. It was found that most of the test subjects felt so much better that they couldn't be considered as being depressed anymore. The most important outcome of

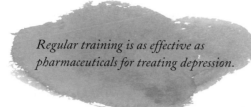

Regular training is as effective as pharmaceuticals for treating depression.

all was that just as many participants in the exercise group got better as those in the group that took Zoloft. In other words, regular physical activity turned out to be as effective as pharmaceuticals in the treatment of depression.

Exercise is healthier over the long term

Despite his study's sensational results, Blumenthal didn't rest on his laurels. He decided to keep track of his test subjects a little more to see if the positive effects of exercise lasted longer than four months. That makes sense, since one emerges from depression in a fragile state, often without realizing it—many feel great and believe that everything is back to normal, even though it's easy to sink back into depression. The ice under our feet is much thinner than we think.

As it happens, fascinating observations were made at a check-in with the people from the three groups six months later. During that time, the participants were not assigned to groups but could choose for themselves what they wanted to do. Some opted for exercise, others chose therapy sessions, and some took medication. Who fared better? Well, those who exercised appeared to be the least likely to relapse: less than one in ten, or 8 percent of the group, became depressed again over that six-month period. On the other hand, the rate of depression in the group who took medication was more than one in three, or 38 percent of the group. Thus, exercise didn't merely provide the same shield against depression as medication; it offered *stronger* protection than medication.

That going for a run should reveal itself to be as effective as a best-selling antidepressant pill, which costs billions to develop, seemed almost too good to be true. Is it indeed the case that exercise produces even *better* results in overcoming depression, over the long term, than medication? Yes, this is exactly what the tests proved. The results were nothing less than astonishing and were, of course, reported on in the papers, but did they garner the same media exposure as the antidepressant medication? No, they got nowhere near the same level of attention.

Billions of dollars have been spent on the marketing of antidepressant pharmaceuticals. In contrast, how much has been spent on spreading the word about how training has the same effect? In all likelihood, very few dollars. Of course, there aren't the same inherent commercial opportunities in that type of information. No one is interested in touting physical activity as widely as a pill that can bring in a lot of money, especially when pharmaceutical marketing budgets are pretty much unlimited. This is why so many people don't know the amazing effect training has on depression.

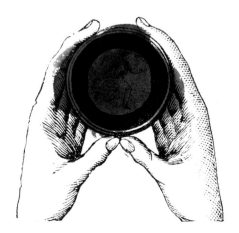

More proof of the benefits of exercise

Blumenthal's results aren't unique. Recently, some scientists decided to compile the papers they could find on exercise that is used in the treatment of depression. There were hundreds of scientific studies from the 1980s onward, from which they selected the top thirty. As many as twenty-five of those studies showed that training provides protection from depression. It's unusual to find such a large set of positive results in these situations. It looks like research has finally caught up and shown in black and white that exercise is an excellent means to treat depression. Even though running seems to produce the best outcome, the compendium of papers indicated that even walking is helpful in preventing it. As little as a twenty- to thirty-minute daily walk can stave off depression and make you feel better!

While the objective of these tests was to see if depression could be treated with physical activity, it was not to find the causes of depression. To discover that reason, we need to look at the substances in the brain that control how we feel: dopamine, serotonin, and noradrenaline.

The brain is not a chemical soup

Serotonin, noradrenaline, and dopamine are substances in the brain that transmit signals between the brain cells—in scientific parlance they're referred to as *neurotransmitters*—and they influence how we feel. Lack of all three neurotransmitters has been connected to depression, and many antidepressant medications are effective by increasing the levels of those neurotransmitters. Selective serotonin reuptake inhibitors (SSRIs), the world's most widely prescribed type of antidepressant medication, raise the level of serotonin; there are also drugs that boost levels of dopamine and noradrenaline. Serotonin, noradrenaline, and dopamine do a lot more than make you feel depressed, or not. They are also essential to the makeup of your personality and important for your cognitive abilities, such as concentration, motivation, and decision making.

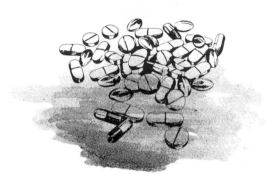

THE DRUGS DO WORK

It's important to emphasize that antidepressant medications do work. They have saved many lives and eased the suffering of millions of people. Anyone who suffers from depression should consider taking medication and seek out professional help.

This is not about using *either* pharmaceuticals *or* training, and it is not advisable for you to discontinue your medication simply because you run or bike on a regular basis. The best effect is achieved if you combine both approaches, since the combination of medication and training is especially powerful. For those who find that medication does not work for them, training might be a good alternative to drugs. Training can also be a good option for people who experience strong side effects of medication.

I want to stress that this book's purpose is not to slam medication, but to show what happens in the brain when we exercise. I'm not in the least worried that there won't be enough people praising the benefits of pharmaceuticals. However, I believe that the effects achieved by exercise and training get way *too little* attention—and that's why I wrote this book.

Serotonin has an inhibitory effect, which modulates the brain's activities. Serotonin calms overactive brain cells and suppresses activity in the entire brain so that worries and anxiety recede. Serotonin creates calm, harmony, and a feeling of inner strength. A lack of serotonin can make you feel fretful and anxious.

Noradrenaline affects how alert, attentive, and focused you are. Low levels of noradrenaline can make you feel tired and down, while too much of it can make you feel keyed up, hyperactive, and unable to settle.

Dopamine is central to the brain's reward system and affects your motivation and your drive. Good food, social interaction, and sex raises dopamine levels, which in turn influences you to try to get more of it. Every little "like" on social media releases a small kick of dopamine, which makes you want to check your cell phone again to see if you've gotten more "likes." All addictive drugs, such as amphetamines, cocaine, and nicotine, raise dopamine levels. Dopamine is also important for concentration and decision making—as you've read in the chapter *Improved concentration*.

It would be very cool if we could draw the conclusion that anyone who is depressed lacks serotonin, noradrenaline, and/or dopamine and replaces what is missing with pills. Sadly, it's not that simple. The image of the brain as a kind of "chemical soup" containing the ingredients serotonin, noradrenaline, and dopamine—in which a lack of one or several causes us to suffer from depression—is too simplistic. There's no way to say for sure if someone is lacking in serotonin, noradrenaline, or dopamine.

One reason is that these substances are interconnected in a larger system of the brain where they don't just affect one another; they also influence a slew of other substances that are pivotal to our well-being. This system is so complex that we have a long way to go before we can fully grasp the extent of it. We should see the brain as an advanced network where activities in different areas mutually affect one another, rather than as a soup of poorly measured ingredients.

Regardless of their complexity, there is no doubt that serotonin, noradrenaline, and dopamine are all central to our feelings—and pharmaceuticals and physical training can raise their levels. The effects of exercise are typically felt *after* a workout and can last anywhere from one to a few hours. If you continue to exercise regularly, these levels will increase over time, not just after training but over the next twenty-four hours. Physical activity can increase serotonin, noradrenaline, and dopamine the same way antidepressant pharmaceuticals do.

THE BRAIN'S MIRACLE MATTER

A great mystery surrounds antidepressant medication. When they're administered to a depressed person, serotonin and dopamine levels usually rise immediately, but without the person feeling any better. It often takes weeks for depression to clear, and the same applies to the effects of physical training. Levels of dopamine and serotonin increase as soon as the first run, but the antidepressant effects don't kick in until after several weeks of regular running.

If serotonin and dopamine play such important roles in how we feel, we should notice their effects immediately, but that's not the case. Perhaps the increase of the two substances, whether by medication or training, is just the first step toward something else that's taking place in the brain, with this "something else" being what makes us feel better in the end. What could it be, then? In neurological research, more and more scientists are looking at what has been dubbed a miracle matter for the brain. Its name is *brain-derived neurotrophic factor* (BDNF).

BDNF is a protein that the brain creates in, among other places, the cerebral cortex (the brain's outer layer) and the hippocampus. We need to be careful when calling something a "miracle," especially in medical research, but the fact is BDNF has such a positive impact on the brain that its moniker is well deserved.

When the brain cells receive BDNF, they acquire protection from things that would otherwise damage or kill them. If we subject brain cells to an oxygen deficit, low blood sugar, an attack of free radicals, or other toxic substances, it typically leads to cell damage or cell death; however, they will be shielded if they get some BDNF first. If someone suffers brain damage—by having a stroke, or taking a hard blow to the head, for instance—the brain seems to pump out BDNF, probably in the effort to save itself. The substance is sent out as a type of brain rescue squad to limit the damage, much like when our white blood cells produce antibodies to fight an infection or when blood platelets coagulate at the site of an injury.

That's how BDNF protects the brain cells. In addition, it oversees the creation of new brain cells and helps these newly formed cells survive their vulnerable early stage. BDNF strengthens the connection between brain cells, which is important for learning and memory. BDNF also makes the brain more flexible and slows the aging of the cells. The list of its benefits is so long it's almost ridiculous. BDNF is, in short, the brain's natural fertilizer. It is as important for the brain's health whether we are children, adults, or elderly.

What does this have to do with depression? Well, BDNF levels appear to be low in people who suffer from depression; this phenomenon has also been observed in the brains of those who have committed suicide. If a sufferer is treated with antidepressants, his or her level of BDNF increases. And the better you feel when recovering from depression, the more BDNF you seem to build up. But that's not all. Levels of BDNF aren't just connected to depression; they also seem to affect our personality traits, as well. Low levels of BDNF appear to be more common in more neurotic people!

Run up the fertilizer levels

Now for the big question: How can we get more of this miraculous product? Can we swallow it in a pill? Unfortunately, no, because it would be

THE *REAL* HAPPY PILL

destroyed by the acid in our stomach. Even if it were possible to protect the BDNF from our stomach acid, it would not make it through the blood-brain barrier. The same would happen if we injected BDNF directly into our bloodstream—the substance would not pass through the blood-brain barrier. Theoretically, one could drill a hole in the skull and inject the BDNF right into it, but who would agree to do that?

However, there is a way to raise the levels of BDNF in a natural way, and it is—*drumroll, please*—exercise! There is *nothing* as effective as physical activity to get the brain to make BDNF. We've seen in animal experiments that the brain immediately starts making this substance when they're physically active, and it continues to do so for a few hours after they have stopped. A great deal of BDNF seems to be generated when the heart's rate is properly elevated. It's also worth keeping up regular training even if the brain starts producing BDNF right after the initial workout, because an identical dose of exercise appears to generate more BDNF per workout as the regimen progresses over time. Let's say you run for thirty minutes twice a week; your brain will slowly produce more and more BDNF with each run, without you having to run longer or faster. If you quit training, the raised levels of BDNF will last for up to two weeks before they start to fall. This means that, from the standpoint of BDNF alone, you don't have to be physically active every single day.

Cardiovascular training is responsible for increased BDNF levels, while strength training doesn't appear to have the same effect. You'll need to exercise aerobically, using interval training, preferably regularly and vigorously, if you wish to generate more BDNF. Elevating the heart rate is important—if not always, then at least from time to time.

Do all roads lead to BDNF?

There are many reasons for becoming depressed or feeling low. Someone might be going through a traumatic event, such as a divorce or a death. Perhaps someone is being subjected to long-term stress. If you walk around for extended periods with high levels of cortisol (the stress hormone) in your body, your risk of becoming depressed rises. Likewise, you can become depressed after a short burst of stress caused by an extremely intense, perhaps life-threatening, event.

But a lot of depression seems to come out of nowhere, and this is something that's being closely monitored today in the effort to understand what might be the root cause. It appears that there could be other reasons for depression besides exterior factors—it could stem from the brain. Somehow, it seems to start from within the body and emerges from unexpected sources. Among other things, being overweight or obese increases one's risk of suffering from depression—not only because the person feels stigmatized or stared at because of their appearance (although this, of course, can be a contributing factor), but also due to something on a purely biological level. One possibility is the fat tissue releases a substance that affects the brain, which can in turn lead to depression. There are several substances under suspicion. Fatty tissue is not just a passive source of energy; it constantly sends signals to the rest of the body to report on existing stocks. These signals are sent with the assistance of different substances, several of which can affect our brain and how we feel.

We're also aware that people with hormonal imbalances, such as the levels of the female hormone estrogen, are at greater risk for depression. Besides, we have a constant, low-grade inflammation in the body, and that too can increase our likelihood of becoming depressed. Some medications inhibit inflammation—anti-inflammatory drugs—appearing to have an effect against depression.

So, depression seems to have many causes. Does this mean there is a common link between obesity, disturbed estrogen levels, inflammation, and the stress hormone cortisol? It looks increasingly like that might be the case, and it boils down to four letters: BDNF. In fact, it seems these disorders can affect BDNF. Stress leads almost immediately to a drop in the production of BDNF. Even carrying too much weight/being

THE MIRACULOUS BACKSTORY OF MIRACLE MATTER

The foundation for the discovery of the brain creating its own fertilizer was laid in the 1930s by the Italian physician and researcher Rita Levi-Montalcini. Being Jewish, she was barred from conducting research by Italy's Fascist regime and lost her position as scientist at the University of Turin. She had to flee several times during WWII, but she never gave up her research. Even though she had neither a position nor a laboratory, she continued her work in her bedroom, at home, using items from her sewing kit as tools.

She used chicken embryos as test subjects for her research into the nervous system. One day, she discovered that something odd had happened in the presence of tumor cells from mice. The nerve cells in the chicken embryo grew at a record pace and in places where they had no place growing at all, such as in blood vessels. The only reasonable explanation for this was that the tumor cells must have secreted a substance that caused rampant growth of the nerve cells. It wasn't until the 1950s that, together with the German professor Viktor Hamburger, she solved the puzzle of the small protein released by the tumor cells: *nerve growth factor* (NGF).

Levi-Montacini soon realized that NGF didn't make all types of nerve cells grow and concluded that there must be several similar substances that could stimulate nerve growth. In the 1980s, another such substance, which showed itself to be closely related to NGF, was discovered. It was given the name *BDNF*—brain-derived neurotrophic factor.

If quick recognition for advances in the field is what you seek, don't go into research. It wasn't until 1986 that Levi-Montalcini was awarded the Nobel Prize in Medicine, in acknowledgement for her great contributions. Rita Levi-Montalcini kept on working every day up into her nineties. She died in 2012 at 103 years of age, and was at the time the oldest living Nobel Prize winner.

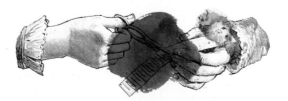

overweight, having impaired estrogen levels, and inflammation can lead to low levels of BDNF, which can make us feel depressed. In other words, BDNF seems to play a central, maybe even pivotal, role in the development of a depression—regardless of its root cause. Knowing this, we should make sure to increase our BDNF levels, and we can do that by exercising. It will help no matter what the cause of the depression.

A disposition that leans toward depression can be partly blamed on genetics, so if a parent has suffered from it, the chances of his or her offspring having it increases. But if some people carry an increased genetic risk, how does that square up with BDNF? Perfectly well, it turns out! BDNF can look a bit different from person to person, and a certain genetic variation is more common among people who suffer from depression. In fact, BDNF is one of the few genes that would be interesting to examine if we want to find the answer as to whether an individual has a genetic predisposition for depression or not.

New brain cells fight depression

The brain tends to shrink a little in a person who suffers from depression. Actually, this happens to everyone. From around the age of twenty-five, the brain's size decreases by about 0.5 percent per year, but it seems to happen more quickly in someone with depression. It is tied to, among other things, the fact that not enough new brain cells are being created. Now we know for sure that new brain cells are created even in adulthood (more about this in the chapter *Jog your memory*), but regeneration is inhibited in someone who suffers from depression.

The current thinking among some scientists is that depression is caused by not having enough new brain cells being generated. Not that the creation of new brain cells is less vigorous due to depression—but that the lack of creation is in fact the reason for the depression. Much points to this hypothesis. If rats are given antidepressants, the amount of newly created brain cells in the hippocampus increases by 50 percent. This doesn't happen overnight; it takes a few weeks for the new cells to form. This is the same amount of time it takes someone who is on anti-depressant medication to begin feeling better. Is this a coincidence? If there is a correlation here, and many things indicate there might be one, it means that antidepressant drugs kick-start the formation of new brain cells and clear the depression.

Medication is not the only thing that can help generate new brain cells; exercise can jump-start the production of new cells in the hippocampus, too. Few things, if any, are as good at firing up the regeneration of brain cells as physical activity. New brain cells aren't just good for those who are depressed; they also play an important role in the brain regardless of how we feel. Even those who are not depressed will benefit from the new cells. So, which substance is responsible for the brain's cell regeneration? You've guessed it: it's BDNF.

Your self-efficacy can cure you

Thus, several things happen in the brain when we become depressed: levels of dopamine, serotonin, noradrenaline, and BDNF fall. Fewer new brain cells are created. Never mind which one of these is the most relevant—we don't know this yet (it's more than likely that they're all linked), but we do know that physical exercise helps.

Aside from the biological impact on the newly created brain cells and on molecules such as dopamine and BDNF, there are other reasons why physical training is a good treatment for depression. One, just like my female patient in the ER, you yourself can get a handle on the situation. You're actively doing something to get well; in my case, the patient started to exercise. In the research community, we talk about *self-efficacy*, which basically means "belief in one's own ability to complete a task or reach a goal." Self-efficacy may sound a bit hollow, but it is in fact an established psychological concept. You increase your self-efficacy with regular training, and you are pleased with yourself. This goes for kids, as well.

Feeling down or being depressed is kind of like being at a mental stand-still, where you are unable to make any progress in life—everything slows down, and the brain doesn't receive as many impressions as before. Moving your body is diametrically opposite to this. Depression is also often recognized in a person if you withdraw, stop socializing with people, and no longer engage in what you used to enjoy doing. Consequently, the brain gets less stimulation and you feel even worse, creating a vicious circle. John Ratey, an American psychiatrist at Harvard University, describes depression as a loss of contact with the sufferer's human connections, as well as the person's brain cells. Engaging in physical activity is one way to break this vicious cycle. You get out, you meet people, and you become less solitary; at the same time, your brain cells break out of their isolation.

These sorts of behavioral changes are often more difficult to measure than, say, levels of dopamine and BDNF, for which you can obtain a measurable number. But just because terms such as *self-efficacy* and *behavior modification* don't sound as objective as "increased levels of dopamine" doesn't mean they are not important.

A more positive personality

The woman I talked about at the beginning of this chapter is just one of many people who have felt much better after starting regular workouts. In her case, as well as the cases of several others, it also seems like their entire personality changed for the better. First, I thought this was just a coincidence. Surely, exercise and training won't transform your *personality*? As a matter of fact, research shows that people who exercise regularly don't just become happier; they also seem to experience small changes in their fundamental personality traits.

Research in Finland, Japan, and South Africa has shown that those who train regularly tend to be less cynical and less neurotic. In addition, they feel a greater rapport with people in their environment. The same exact pattern was observed in Holland when they examined close to twenty thousand pairs of twins. Those who exercised twice a week were more socially open and less neurotic.

108

The answer to which came first—the chicken or the egg—is of course not obvious. Training could make a person less cynical and less neurotic; it might also just as easily mean that people who are cynical and neurotic don't exercise as much. What can vouch for training affecting personality is that we're gradually beginning to understand the role of molecules in certain personality traits.

Serotonin and dopamine aren't just important in how you feel; the variations in levels of those substances in individual people probably contribute to our differences in personality. Dopamine, for example, has been linked to curiosity and a willingness to try new experiences, while serotonin is linked to compromise, and also to how neurotic a person is.

Boiling personality down to molecules and mental processes is not easy. The biology that determines your personality and how you feel is tremendously complex. By the same token, it is just biology. Even if these two neurotransmitters can't begin to explain your entire personality, they still play a part in it. The fact that dopamine and serotonin levels are influenced, over the short and long term, by exercise means that it is not unreasonable at all to suppose that training can affect personality.

Training becomes a drug

One of exercise's effects on how we feel is more extreme than others. It's a fact that we can feel completely high from moving our bodies, in which case exercise becomes a sort of endogenous drug. I am talking, of course, about what is commonly known as *runner's high*, which you might have experienced at some point yourself. You should not chase runner's high if you're suffering from depression, but it still deserves a mention in a book such as this. The story of what it is, and what causes it, is nothing short of thrilling.

The hunt for the mystical morphine

It has been known for over two thousand years that opium can blot out pain and cause euphoria. The dried sap from the opium poppy, from which opium is made, was used as medicine and as a popular drug during the Roman Empire. At the start of the nineteenth century, German scientists managed to isolate morphine, the active ingredient in opium, and began using it in healthcare situations, most notably as a painkiller for wounded soldiers. It proved to be amazingly effective. Even when soldiers had lost their arms or legs, small doses in increments weighing tenths of a gram could almost knock out all their pain. It was incredible that such a low dose could have that deep an impact, especially when compared to alcohol, which can also dull pain, but only in doses hundreds of times larger to achieve a similar effect.

At the beginning of the 1970s, it was discovered that there is a type of receptor on the brain cells' surface that morphine binds to, which explains why the drug is so powerful. This raised the question of why these receptors even existed. Did nature want us to turn into morphine addicts? That doesn't seem likely; a more plausible reason was that the brain could produce its own morphine-like substance, and that the receptors were meant for this self-made and still-unknown substance.

Scientists all over the world raced to identify the brain's own morphine, and those efforts quickly produced results. In 1974, it was discovered that pigs' brains released a mysterious substance; it appeared that the animal's own brain produced a substance that had a structure similar to morphine's. That same year, an American psychiatrist made the same discovery when he examined calves' brains. The mysterious substances found in the pigs and calves, which were closely related, turned out to be a "self-morphine." This substance, which exists even in humans, received the name *endogenous morphine*—morphine originating from the body. However, it became known by a shorter name: *endorphins*.

Endorphins, like morphine, are incredibly effective at suppressing pain. And just like morphine, they can produce feelings of euphoria. But why would the brain reward itself with a dose of morphine? Why does this mechanism exist, and when does the brain reward itself? The question was raised as to whether there was a natural

110

circumstance in which human beings experience pain relief and euphoria simultaneously, without the help of medication or drugs.

One such state is explained by the American long-distance runner James Fixx in his best-selling book *The Complete Book of Running*. Sometimes when Fixx was running long distances, he experienced a feeling of euphoria and pain relief that he called *runner's high*. Turns out he was far from alone in experiencing runner's high, and reports soon came in from other athletes who participated in different types of aerobic training. Swimmers, cyclists, and rowers had all felt the same sensation but had simply called it by different names. Rowers called it, appropriately enough, *rower's high*.

Run yourself high!

Jame Fixx's book came out during the running craze of the 1970s, and runner's high soon became a buzzword. It was widely accepted that the newly discovered endorphins were at the crux of this effect. Today, most runners know about runner's high, though not many have experienced it. The effect is so much stronger than simply feeling a bit more alert—runner's high is the most extreme impact physical training can have on our mood.

I, myself, have felt it twice, and it's impossible to explain the feeling other than to say that it's pure magic! It's not the same type of calm you feel at the end of a workout. No, it's more akin to the euphoria of when all pain disappears, all impressions become more intense, and you feel like you could run forever and ever, as fast as the wind. The feeling is so intense that you will most definitely remember it if you ever experience it. If you're unsure if you've felt runner's high—it's more than likely that you haven't.

It seems logical that it's the endorphins that are behind this feeling, because it is so reminiscent of the effect of morphine. However, the source of runner's high is still being debated, and some scientists believe that there's more to this happy state than just endorphins. To shed some light on the issue, a few scientists in Munich, Germany, decided to examine the brains of runners in their local runners' club. They measured the level of endorphins with a PET scan before and two hours after a high-speed run. The results were unambiguous: all the runners had lots of endorphins after the run, especially in their prefrontal cortex and limbic systems, the two areas in the brain central to controlling feelings. When the runners rated their levels of euphoria, it was obvious that the more euphoria the runner reported feeling, the more endorphins were present in the brain.

This is where the debate on what causes runner's high could have ended, but there are a few counterarguments against the notion that endorphins are the lone reason for this feeling. First, endorphin molecules are big, which would make it difficult for them to break the blood-brain barrier. Second, when long-distance runners were given a substance to block morphine, and thus by extension endorphins, runners could still feel runner's high.

Are highs only caused by endorphins?

Another possibility is that runner's high is caused by endocannabinoids. Like endorphins, they are a type of painkilling substance produced by the body; however, they are smaller than endorphins and can therefore make their way into the brain more easily. Like in the case of endorphins, there are specific receptors for endocannabinoids on the brain cells that addictive drugs can bind to. (Endocannabinoids use the same receptors in the brain as the active ingredient in hashish and marijuana.)

The suggestion that endocannabinoids might have something to do with runner's high was bolstered when French scientists genetically modified mice so they lacked endocannabinoid receptors. The rodents' desire to move subsequently changed. Normally, it's enough that mice in a cage have access to a wheel to make them run of their own volition. However, the genetically modified mice didn't care to move at all and only ran half as much as mice typically do. The extent to which

112

a mouse can experience euphoria and runner's high is difficult to assess, but it has been possible to see that levels of endocannabinoids increase in humans after they have run. Walking is not enough; one must run for at least forty-five to sixty minutes. This fits with what's required to reach a runner's high—by definition, it cannot be achieved by walking.

Some scientists believe that aside from endorphins and endocannabinoids, running increases levels of dopamine and serotonin. Others believe that it's linked to body temperature and that we become euphoric as we heat up. The most plausible explanation is that runner's high doesn't rely on one lone factor but several of them, and that endorphins and endocannabinoids both contribute to it. Whatever the biological source may be, it is mostly of interest to scientists. Otherwise, for runners, cyclists, and tennis players—or whatever else we do when we're physically active—it's enough to know that runner's high happens, not why it happens.

Our heritage from the savanna

Becoming euphoric by running is probably a leftover effect from our ancestors' life on the savanna. No doubt, some had to run long distances while hunting, a method that Australian aborigines and the Kalahari Desert's bushmen still use. When you stalked prey for several miles to tire it out, it was important not to give up the chase, which is when endorphins came in handy. If you twisted your ankle or your muscles ached, endorphins blotted out the pain, and when the going got tough, that feeling of euphoria made it easier to keep going. This increased the likelihood of a kill, which is probably why we still experience runner's high, even today.

There is quite a lot of evidence indicating that runner's high may be a natural way to get us to keep running and catch our food. It has been shown that if we decrease our level of body fat, levels of leptin—a hormone that is released by fat—decreases, which sounds the alarm that energy levels are dropping and need to be topped up. Our body doesn't want us to be skinny, quite the opposite, in fact. It wants us to carry around a substantial reserve of energy. If this hypothesis is correct—that we need a shot of pleasure to keep up the strength to continue searching for food—then our body is letting us know, via runner's high: "Your stores of energy are soon depleted—don't give up, keep moving and find more food!" To help us along, it makes us feel euphoric.

How do you achieve a runner's high?

We know that you must run for at least forty-five minutes, and the more you run, the bigger the chance of feeling a runner's high. The brain appears to give itself ever-increasing doses of endorphins the more you train. Consequently, the likelihood of feeling a runner's high increases over time, so don't give up! However, there are no guarantees, because not everyone will get to feel it.

It has been shown that your pain threshold increases when you've been running for a while—the same as with morphine. By sticking people with a needle or pinching them to test their tolerance to pain, we've noticed that it takes more for you to feel pain during running than if the pain threshold was tested at rest. This supports the idea that endorphins not only make us feel euphoria, but also provide pain relief. And there is no doubt that pain relief can be powerful: it has been calculated that the endorphins felt during high-speed running is equal to a ten-milligram shot of morphine, a commonly administered dose for an arm or leg fracture. That's why we sometimes see runners continually running even when they have stress fractures (caused by long-term overuse and repetitive motions). They don't feel the pain so long as they run, though it flares up the moment they stop and the effect of the endorphins wears out. While runner's high is exercise's most extreme effect on the brain, your well-being will improve even if you don't feel a dramatic rush of endorphins. Anyone who exercises is rewarded with endorphins and endocannabinoids, even if they don't reach runner's high.

114

THE RIGHT PRESCRIPTION TO FEEL BETTER OVERALL

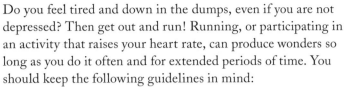

Do you feel tired and down in the dumps, even if you are not depressed? Then get out and run! Running, or participating in an activity that raises your heart rate, can produce wonders so long as you do it often and for extended periods of time. You should keep the following guidelines in mind:

Run three times a week, about thirty to forty minutes each time. The intensity should be at least 70 percent of your VO_2 max. Keeping a normal speed works well, but you should still feel winded and break a sweat.

Biking or any other type of cardiovascular training is a good substitute for running. It's the intensity and the length of time that count, not what you do or where you do it.

Keep this up for at least three weeks! It's true that many feel better after exercising just once, but to feel better during the day and not just after a workout, you need to train regularly over several weeks. Don't expect too many results in the first weeks.

IF YOU SUFFER FROM DEPRESSION

Training is as effective as medication for mild or nonclinical depressive conditions, but you must run (or partake in an equivalent type of exercise) three times a week, and for forty-five minutes each time. It takes about six weeks to notice some changes, so don't give up!

Medication works best for clinical depression and suicidal thinking. It's not realistic to expect the sufferer to begin exercising as treatment, since it might take all their strength just to get out of bed. *Always* speak to your physician, and *never* quit your medication on your own!

It's not a question of *either-or* here. Training is good. Medication is good. The ideal is a combination of both. Regular exercise and physical activity could also help prevent future depressive episodes. You become more resilient to stress, which is the most common cause of depression. Everything is connected!

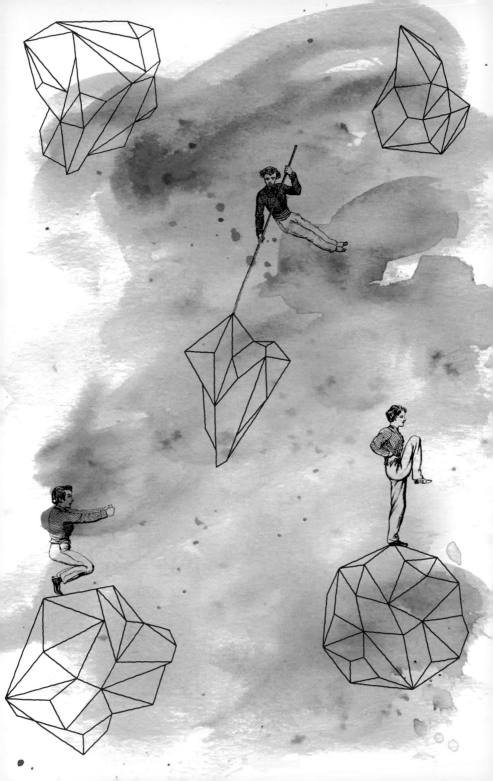

5. JOG YOUR MEMORY

Take care of all your memories.
For you cannot relive them.
BOB DYLAN

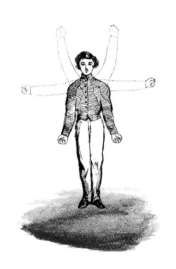

I n the mid-1990s, a group of scientists decided to see which part of the brain is most affected by exercise. They already had a theory before the study began: the cerebral cortex and the cerebellum (situated where the spinal cord meets the brain) are both important for coordination of physical movement, so it seemed natural that these areas would be the most affected by physical activity, just as running has more influence on cardiovascular fitness than on muscular strength.

The starting point was to see which part of the brain creates the most BDNF (the brain's own miracle medication I described in the chapter *The real happy pill*) in mice that run in a wheel in their cage. The strange thing was that when the mice brains were examined, it was revealed that it was neither the cortex nor the cerebellum that produced the most BDNF, but the hippocampus—the brain's memory center. This discovery became one of the most important clues as to why exercise has such a huge effect on memory. Over the past decade, research on animals and humans has proved that our memory is strengthened by physical activity. In fact, nothing seems to be more important for our memory than physical activity.

STOP YOUR BRAIN FROM SHRINKING

rain shrinks throughout life, and unfortunately this process s much earlier than most of us would like. The brain is at its largest when we're about twenty-five years old, after which it gets a little smaller every passing year. Certainly, new brain cells are created throughout our lifetime, but cells die more quickly than new ones are generated. The net effect is that we lose approximately one hundred thousand brain cells per second every twenty-four hours. This goes on constantly. Year-round. Even if there are plenty of cells to glean from—the brain contains about a hundred billion cells—the loss will become noticeable over time. Over one year, the brain's volume will decrease by between 0.5 and 1 percent.

The memory center, the hippocampus—big as a thumb and shaped like a seahorse—is one of the areas of the brain that shrinks as we age. We have two hippocampi, one on each side of the brain, and they are located deep inside each temporal lobe. Its size decreases by about 1 percent each year. Those slowly but steadily shrinking hippocampi are why our memory gets worse as years go by.

For a long time, we thought that the brain's development could only be adversely—never positively—impacted by such things as alcohol and drugs, which accelerate the brain's aging and hasten the shrinking of the hippocampus. To stop this development, or to even turn it around, was considered impossible. It is against this backdrop that we will now see some of the most convincing evidence of the amazing effect exercise and physical training have not only on memory, but on the brain as a whole. American scientists used MRI scans to examine the brains of 120 individuals and to measure their hippocampi at two different times, with one gap year in between. The test subjects were randomly assigned to two groups that performed two different types of activities. One group did endurance training while the other engaged in mellow exercises like stretching that did not raise their heart rates.

One year later, the members of the group who trained had become fitter, in contrast to the other group's members who had performed the gentler exercises. Nothing surprising so far, but what had happened to the hippocampus? The hippocampi in people who had done the soft exercises had shrunk by 1.4 percent, which was no surprise either, since the hippocampus does shrink by about 1 percent each year after all.

What was very interesting was that the hippocampus didn't shrink at all in the members of the group that had endurance-trained; in fact, it had *grown* and become larger by 2 percent. Instead of aging by one year, the hippocampus had rejuvenated itself and size-wise had become two years younger! And that's not all: the fitter the test subjects had gotten, the larger their hippocampi had grown. Among those who had seen the greatest improvement in their fitness, the hippocampus had grown by more than 2 percent.

Of course, this raises the very important question of how this happened. One not unreasonable hypothesis is that the brain's fertilizer, BDNF (which increases as we become more physically active), played a role. Perhaps you remember from the chapter *The* real *happy pill* that BDNF can strengthen the bond between brain cells and can therefore influence how well we remember things. And quite rightly so: when the scientists examined the levels of BDNF, they noticed that the more they had increased, the more the hippocampus had grown.

What miraculous training program could revitalize and promote regrowth of such an important part of the brain in a single year? Did the test subjects pedal away on stationary bikes like bats out of hell, or did they run at draconian intervals? Not at all. The truth is that they neither biked nor ran. The only exercise they engaged in was a forty-minute power walk, three times a week. This means that you can stop, and perhaps even reverse, your brain's aging and strengthen your memory by power walking or running a few times a week!

However, it's always better to be cautious in drawing conclusions when reading about these kinds of tests. Experiments are one thing, reality is another. If the hippocampus can be protected from aging, or even rejuvenated and grown bigger, what does that mean for us in life? Do we truly see improvement in our memory just by being physically active? The short answer is: Yes, absolutely!

120

A long history of past tests points very clearly in the same direction: both short- and long-term memory are improved through exercise, and the gradual breakdown of the hippocampus that goes with aging can be slowed down, and even reversed.

Genetic rejuvenation of the brain

As if it weren't enough that exercise safeguards the hippocampus from age-related shrinkage, it appears that it also offers protection against genetic aging. Just like other cells in the brain and the body, the hippocampus contains our genetic material. Our entire DNA and all our genes can be found in every brain cell. Normally genes don't change during our lifetime, but our *use* of them changes, which can cause the body's organs, including the brain, to age.

If we examine the hippocampus brain cells of mice at different ages, we'll find that in one group of genes the changes follow the animals' aging. Among other things, these genes control the growth of brain cells and their ability to create connections to one another. As the mice age, the genes become less active, and this gradual genetic change doesn't just make the hippocampus age—it also makes the entire brain grow older.

However, not even cells' aging at the genetic level means that we're doomed with no recourse. When the test animals are allowed to run on a treadmill, something happens that can only be described as a miracle. Many of the genes that are adversely affected by aging are also influenced by training—in a positive way. Through mechanisms that are not yet fully understood, the hippocampus cells appear to become genetically younger after the test animals have run.

These effects are powerful, but not instantaneous. The mice ran daily for eight weeks, which for us would be the equivalent of exercising regularly for several years—this means that the occasional jog is not enough. But intriguingly, it seems that those who are patient and who remain physically active regularly over a long time not only grow a larger hippocampus, but are also rewarded with revitalized hippocampus cells.

PRACTICAL MEMORY TRAINING

How do we go about strengthening memory with physical activity? Do we need to keep at it for several months, or do we notice any effects right away? Does it work best *before* learning something, or is it better to exercise *after* learning?

You don't have to work very long in the beginning to notice an effect. It has been shown that three months of regular endurance training leads to significant improvement in the ability to recall words. And it's worth putting in the effort, because *how* much better your memory gets (i.e., the number of words you remember) is connected to how much fitter you become. Those who improved their fitness the most also saw the most benefit to their memory. This link is especially interesting, considering that the hippocampus grows larger as we get fitter.

Do you think that three months is a long time? Don't worry, you'll notice results faster than that. Healthy individuals who biked regularly on stationary bikes were compared to a group of people of similar ages who did not cycle. Before the test began, the cyclists and noncyclists had comparable results on several different memory tests. However, the cyclists soon pulled ahead in both fitness and memory. Six weeks in, it was obvious that the group that cycled were better at the memory tests, and the differences became more substantial the longer the study lasted. The cyclists' memory kept improving, while the noncyclists stayed in one spot, both in terms of fitness and memory.

When the cyclists' brains were studied with MRI, the scans revealed that improved memory went hand in hand with increased blood flow to the hippocampus, our memory center. This increased blood flow would certainly explain why the hippocampus works better. Interestingly, it looks like the blood flow increases first, after which memory improves.

An instant memory boost

Are you as impatient as I am and feel that six weeks is way too long to see progress? The truth is training improves memory immediately!

122

*If you want to boost your memory, train while
you learn something.*

It has been observed that those who did best on the test were those who trained right *before* the test. Moderately fit people who train right before a memory test typically do better than fit people who haven't trained beforehand, illustrating that training has an immediate effect on memory.

But if you'd like to boost your memory to the max, you will need to move and learn at the same time—studying while walking on a treadmill, for instance. This is good to keep in mind even if it may not always be possible to do, of course.

We don't know why individuals who learn something while they exercise remember things better. What probably happens is that the blood flow in the brain increases when you move, the same way blood circulation increases in muscles. This blood flow boost is instantaneous, and when the brain gets more blood, memory works better.

Don't work out to the point of failure

Boosting your memory through exercise doesn't mean it's just a marginal effect that can be measured only in scientific experiments; on the contrary, you will notice these effects. In word tests that measure word recall, it has been shown that you can learn up to 20 percent more words if you're physically active before or while you learn the words, compared to when you are at rest. Those of you who are studying for an exam or who need to learn material for work should think twice before deciding you don't have time for a walk. That walk is probably time well spent.

From a memory standpoint, walking or light jogging is enough to achieve the best effect. However, if you work out to the point of failure and end up exhausted, you run the risk of remembering *less*. Muscles require so much blood that blood flow to the brain decreases slightly, which may be why your memory doesn't work as well. Besides, if you train hard, the brain seems to focus on your movement and not on what you're trying to learn. For example, if you run fast while listening to something you need to remember, your brain is going to focus on running, not on what you hear.

Can running make me a better piano player?

Our memory is not all about learning words, reading texts, or remembering what we did last week. We also have a motor memory for movements, like when we learn to hit a forehand in tennis or play a piano piece. The basis for all learning is that new connections are created among brain cells, which makes you wonder if the conditions for learning a motor skill improve if you exercise. Naturally, your forehand gets better if you practice only that movement. Does this mean that your ability to master the forehand will improve if you run first? Or that biking can improve your ability to learn to play the piano?

To gauge how physical activity influences our motor memory, subjects were asked to play a simple computer game using a joystick to follow a point moving across a screen. The game, which seems simplistic, activates many areas of the brain and is occasionally used in research to measure motor ability.

For this test, subjects were first required to run or bike and then proceed to the computer game. Then they were asked play the game again after some time had passed to see if they improved. Just as your forehand improves with practice, you naturally improve at playing a computer game after some practice. But here's what was noteworthy: when tested, those who had been physically active prior to playing the game were better at it. To be clear: the only difference was that some of the test subjects exercised before the game, and there were no variations in the time spent practicing the game. Nonetheless, those who exercised did better. Some aspect of movement in and of itself helped them to learn to play the game better without having to spend more time practicing.

How then can physical activity make us perform better at motor activities? We can only speculate, but in the minutes to twenty-four hours following the acquisition of a new skill, *memory consolidation* happens. This means that the memory, whether of learning a piano piece or a computer game, is transferred from short-term memory to long-term memory. Let's say you play a simple tune on the piano a few times. You rest for one minute, and then play the tune again. You'll probably remember it quite well as it sits in your short-term memory. But how well will you remember that tune tomorrow? That depends on how strongly the memory has been imprinted, or consolidated, as a long-term memory.

The hippocampus is important in how memories get transferred from short-term to long-term status. As we've seen, exercise makes the hippocampus cells pump out BDNF, which reinforces the connection among brain cells. If we engage in physical activity before learning, BDNF will be pumped out while the memory changes from short term to long term. The conditions for that memory to go into long-term storage will probably improve, since the transmission from short-term to long-term status happens not within minutes of learning something, but more like *twenty-four hours* afterward. This corresponds quite closely to what the computer game test revealed, which is that exercise starts having an effect one day after learning.

This means you will probably become a better piano player if you're physically active before you practice your piano scales! And it signifies that you'll increase your chances of learning that golf swing if you go for a run or a bike ride before heading out on the golf course. Through exercise, you can strengthen your brain's memory during that crucial phase when the memory of the piano piece or golf swing—or whatever skill

125

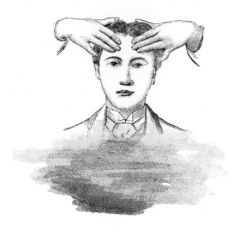

MENTAL PATHS

Basically, our memories are a cluster of brain cells connected to one another. When we experience something new (i.e., create a new memory), new connections called *synapses* are created. These connections don't mean that the cells physically touch one another, but that an end terminal sends a chemical message between them. Nobel Prize winner Santiago Ramón y Cajal described it poetically as "brain cells holding hands," even though cells don't actually touch.

How hard cells hold on to one another depends on how many times they make contact. If you learn a new phone number, a new contact will be created. Each time you dial that number the contact will strengthen—the cells hold on tighter to one another—and you'll remember the number much better each time you dial it. Perhaps you remember that "Neurons that fire together wire together!" On the other hand, if you only learn the phone number once, you will forget it. The connection will weaken if it isn't reinforced, and the brain cells lose the connection.

Similarly, we can look at memories as mental paths that are created among the brain's cells. Well-trodden paths stay put,

126

and so that memory remains. Paths that were recently walked on a few times will grow over and disappear. Some things create a well-worn path right away that embeds itself as a memory for life.

A unique or an unusually intense experience can leave a lifelong mental imprint, even if the path was only "walked on" once. This applies especially to emotionally charged events that have negative connotations, such as threats or danger. Those types of memories are very important from a survival standpoint, and consequently they have priority in the memory bank. Evolutionarily speaking, it's critical to remember what is dangerous so you can avoid it in the future. This means that if you witness something horrible or experience a life-threatening situation, you will most likely remember the event in detail for the rest of your life. Other things that are not as unique or charged, like tying your shoe laces, won't leave a path. The cells hold on to one another for a short while, and then they let go. You'll quickly forget what you did.

Bearing this in mind, you can see how physical activity may contribute to mental paths being well-worn and to cells "holding hard on to one another." As you'll recall from the beginning of this chapter, exercise causes brain cells in the hippocampus to pump out more of the substance called BDNF. BDNF will strengthen the connection among brain cells so they "hold hands even harder," which, to continue with that analogy, means that the mental path becomes well-worn faster. The memory becomes stronger, and, consequently, we remember what we're doing. We remember better, and we learn better.

Physical activity increases levels of BDNF, which in turn reinforces the connections among the brain's cells, making it probably one of the most important reasons why exercise is so beneficial for memory.

you wish to learn—is being saved to long-term memory. The brain cells' ability to create strong and lasting connections between one another increases, and it seems to apply to situations where you are acquiring a language or a motor skill.

Does too much training impair memory?

From the brain's perspective, it's debatable whether more exercise is always better—if you can have too much of a good thing. Is a grueling race such as the Ironman Triathlon, during which participants remain active for ten to twelve continuous hours, good for memory and the brain? We don't know for sure yet, but there is a lot to suggest that such a big effort is more damaging than beneficial to the brain and for memory—at least in the short term.

By selecting from a large pool of mice, American scientists were able to breed specimens that were obsessed with running: those that ran the most could mate, and the offspring that moved the most were in turn allowed to mate. The scientists continued in this manner until they had produced mice that would, of their own free will, run almost three times as much as regular mice. In fact, these ultra-runner mice ran the equivalent of many miles a day for a human being.

The mice's memory was then tested by letting them try out a new maze. Normally, mice that run are quicker to find their way around a new space, since exercise improves memory. However, the ultra-runner mice took much longer than normal to learn the new maze. Their memory was worse, and their blood had high levels of the stress hormone cortisol, which is central to the body's stress response. Cortisol levels typically drop after we've been physically active, so the mice that ran regularly should have had less stress. Instead, these ultra-runner mice seemed to be chronically stressed out.

We don't know for certain yet if this carries over to humans, but it looks like there is a degree at which exercise becomes too much to handle for the brain. At this point, the stress response no longer decreases

> *A walk or a thirty-minute run is enough exercise for boosting memory; it's probably better than running for several hours.*

but *increases,* and memory becomes poorer. Currently we don't know exactly where that stress cut-off is—it probably varies from person to person. However, one conclusion that could possibly be drawn is that anyone who participates in ultra-marathons or similar events should not do so with the intention of strengthening their brain and improving their memory, since they may in fact suffer the opposite outcome. A long walk or a thirty-minute run is plenty for the brain—it's probably much better than running for several hours.

YOUR BRAIN CAN CREATE NEW CELLS

At the dawn of the 1900s, most scientists agreed that the adult brain could not generate any new cells. If we cut ourselves, the cut heals over and new skin cells are produced. Likewise, new hair cells and blood cells form continually. Most of the body's organs are capable of regenerating cells, but nobody thought this to be true about the brain, the explanation being that the brain, comprised of its one hundred billion cells, is so incredibly complex that newly generated cells in an adult brain could not fit in together with the cells originating from birth. It seemed as improbable as thinking you could dismantle a computer, randomly plug in a few circuit boards, and hope the computer would run better. This belief is why many of us were taught in school that the brain we have at twenty years of age is the one we must make do with for the rest of our lives. I remember it being said that if you take a swig of alcohol, you'll lose fifty thousand brain cells that you'll never see again.

"The truth" that was not true at all

We all know that it doesn't hurt to question established "truths" from time to time. In the mid-1990s, some scientists in California decided to take a good look at the question of whether the adult brain can produce new cells. They didn't start off by examining human brains, focusing on those of mice instead. The first question they wanted to clear up was if anything would happen in the brain if the animals were removed from their boring, sterile cages and got more stimulation in what scientists call an *enriched environment*. The mice lived for one month in a cage with plenty of tunnels to hide in, wheels to run on, and toys to play with. They also had the company of more mice. This was indisputably a far more fun environment than the sterile cages the mice were used to. The scientists knew that a change of environment with new experiences could create new connections among the mice's brain cells, because connections are created when we learn something new. But could it affect the animals' brains in some other way? It did indeed!

The new, stimulating environment had a huge effect in the brain—it created lots of new cells. Part of the hippocampus had grown, and the results were dramatic. The number of cells had increased by 15 percent in a few short weeks, which was sensational.

This couldn't be explained by the mice's young age, because the same thing occurred when they performed an identical experiment on older mice. The animals' brains didn't just generate new cells; they seemed to work better. When the mice's memory was tested by lowering them into a pool in which they had to find a hidden platform, the mice who had stayed in the enriched environment located the platform faster. They also had better memory than the mice that spent their days in a sterile cage.

What exactly caused this effect?

This discovery brought up stunning implications. Could this also apply to people who were put in a more stimulating environment? Did this mean that a change of environment and new experiences such as travel, a career

130

change, or a new social circle could lead the brain to create new cells? Could such experiences improve our memory, and perhaps even make us smarter?

First, let's back up a step. What was it in the mice's environment that made their brain create more cells? Was it the toys and the tunnels where they could hide, or was it that there were many other mice around? Or could it have had something to do with the wheel they were running on?

Had it been my guess, I would have ventured that it was a combination of all the factors. Turns out, I was wrong. When the mice *only* ran on the wheel and didn't have access to any other stimulus in their crate, the impact in their brain was widespread. It appears that physical activity—running on the wheel—was the principal factor in the creation of new brain cells. Other stimuli, from toys and tunnels or friends, appeared to have little or no effect.

Finding out that regular running produces so many new brain cells had significant repercussions for several of the scientists. One of them, geneticist Fred "Rusty" Gage, told of how his colleagues had turned their lifestyles around completely and begun running as soon as they saw all the new cells in the mice's brains. They reasoned that if it works in mice, it probably works in humans, too.

But were Gage and his colleagues correct in inferring that the adult human brain could generate new brain cells? This is a difficult question to answer, because it would require studying the brain under a microscope, since a CT scan or MRI cannot provide any clues. In fact, what is needed is an autopsy of a human brain. Even if someone agreed to donate their brain in the name of research after their death, there would still be a problem: How do you figure out if the brain cells are new? It's extremely challenging to tell the difference between old and new brain cells.

Even adults generate new brain cells

The solution came when Peter Eriksson, a Swedish neuroscientist, had a brilliant idea. Oncologists use a substance called *bromodeoxyuridine* (BrdU) to decide whether cancer cells divide and whether the cancer

DO YOU FORGET PAIN?

I've heard the lament "Never again" many times from marathon runners who have just crossed the finish line. And yet, a few weeks later, there they are, signing up for another race. How is it that you can go through a race that you consider intolerably difficult and still choose to line up at starting blocks year after year? A possible explanation is that runners forget how exhausting the event was.

Selective forgetfulness is not some pseudopsychological term, but a medical reality that happens at times such as after childbirth. When a comparison was made between the pain women experienced during labor, at the moment, and the pain they felt after gynecological surgery, it showed that those who had given birth and those who had had surgery rated the pain at about the same intensity. In these cases, the pain of childbirth appears to be comparable to that of a surgical operation.

But when you ask those women to think back and remember the event and the pain a few months later, it turns out that the women who gave birth no longer remember how traumatic it was (at least, not to the same degree). However, those who had undergone surgery remembered the pain as vividly as the day it was performed. Indeed, some women forget how painful it is to give birth. It's one thing to remember that it is painful, but another to remember the *intensity* of that pain. From a biological perspective, this isn't so strange, because if there's one thing that's

132

vital for our species, it's procreation—making more people. That's why it makes sense that we have a natural mechanism that helps us forget labor pain, or in any case for not remembering the pain in so much detail as to not want to give birth again.

The same thing appears to happen with hard physical exertion. When marathon runners who just crossed the finish line graded the pain they felt throughout the race, the average answer was 5.5 on a scale of 10. When they thought back to that race and graded their pain again three to six months later, their answer went down to a 3. They seemed to have forgotten just how painful it was!

Certainly, selective memory is reasonable from a biological perspective. If we remember how hard it was to follow our kill over long distances, it may discourage us from hunting. However, if we forget how tiring it was, we'll be eager to hunt again, increasing our chances of getting food and, in the long run, of survival. This is a likely explanation for our memory's ability to selectively forget the pain inherent in physical activities.

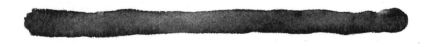

grows. In fact, BrdU can tag new cells—not just cancer cells, but other types of cells, as well. Eriksson realized that if new brain cells were present, BrdU would be able to tag them, too, making it possible to pick them out in the brain samples of deceased cancer patients.

The researchers obtained permission to examine the brains of five deceased patients to look for new cells. Their brains offered a unique insight into the question of whether the brain regenerates throughout life, one of neuroscience's biggest conundrums. It was hoped that, upon examination, the samples would reveal new brain cells marked with BrdU in at least one of the five donors. They found cells in all five of them, and in exactly the same area of the brain as the new cells they found in the mice—the hippocampus.

Incredibly, it was possible to ascertain that the new brain cells were only about a month old, meaning that they had formed while the donor was dying from a serious illness. The brain had still kept on creating new brain cells! It was also visible through the microscope that the new cells had made connections with older brain cells and appeared to have integrated in the hippocampus, meaning they had assimilated into their new environment. It's likely that they functioned and were useful while the patient was still alive.

The significance of the donors' brains containing newly created brain cells was enormous. The news that *neurogenesis*—the creation and development of new nervous tissue—happens even in adults was a sensation, and it made the headlines in newspapers all over the world. Textbooks in the medical field had to be rewritten. The "truth" that brain cells can't regenerate over a lifetime was proven to be false.

However, as is so often the case in the world of scientific research, one answered question usually begets additional unresolved issues. Now the big question was: Does regeneration of cells happen at the same rate no matter how you live your life, and if not, what is it influenced by? Is it possible to speed up this regeneration, and if so, how? One reasonable area of focus would be the influence of physical activity, since studies have already shown how activity produces the best results with mice.

So, is this it? Do we know for sure that exercise leads to a higher rate of brain cell regeneration, even in humans? And do we improve our memory by being physically active? The answer to both those questions is yes. At least, that is the conclusion reached after two decades of research conducted since the discovery of human neurogenesis.

Earlier atom testing could solve the question

Before we continue, let's ask the following question: How important is the regeneration of new brain cells in the hippocampus? Is it only important to scientists? Is it something that is only visible in laboratory experiments but lacks practical significance? To start, regeneration of brain cells is far from insignificant. Approximately one-third of all the cells in the hippocampus are swapped out for new cells over our lifetime.

One can wonder, how are we to know this? When the brain of a deceased person is examined, you can't tell if the cells were made when the person was an adult or if they were present throughout his or her lifetime. The methods used by Fred Gage and Peter Eriksson only showed if the cells had been created recently—after the BrdU was introduced.

To solve this mystery, scientists at Sweden's Karolinska Institute used something that we might not immediately associate with neuroscience: test detonations of atomic weapons.

A lot of blasts were performed during the Cold War of the 1950s and 1960s, many of them in the far-flung islands in the Pacific Ocean. Even though the tests took place on the other side of the globe, the radioactive isotope C-14 got into the atmosphere and spread throughout the world. The concentration of C-14 in the atmosphere has been measured regularly, making it possible to see how much of it has been in the air over the years.

What does this have to do with brain cells? Well, every time a new brain cell is generated, new DNA is created, and C-14 of the same concentration as was present in the atmosphere the year the cell was generated is built right into the DNA's helix. This means you can date a cell if you know the atmosphere's concentration of C-14 over the years. A brain cell that is forty-five years old in a forty-five-year-old man will have been there since the man's birth, while a brain cell that is thirty years old would have been created when the man was a teenager.

Using this method, we can date hippocampus cells in deceased donors who were about ninety years old when they passed away. We can calculate how many cells were the same age as the donor, and how many were younger. The result showed that almost a third of the cells had such concentrations of C-14 in their DNA, indicating that they must have been created after birth. In fact, the tests show that 1,400 new cells are generated in the hippocampus of an adult brain every day. This means that every second of every hour of every day of your adult life, a new cell is created in your hippocampus.

New cells are important for our well-being

Research hasn't only been able to show that large numbers of new cells are created in the hippocampus over your entire life. We now know that regeneration of cells not only strengthens memory, but is also pivotal to our mental well-being. Many believe that depression is an illness caused by poor nerve cell regeneration, and that the lack of new cells is the true cause of depression, as we touched on in the chapter *The* real *happy pill.*

A clue to this hypothesis is that antidepressant medication boosts the regeneration of brain cells. If you block the brain's ability to create new cells in animals, it will render the antidepressants useless and the depression will not clear. In other words, a person may become unresponsive to antidepressants if the brain can't create new cells. This strongly suggests that regeneration of brain cells is critical to our sense of well-being and our ability to recover from a depression. If our ability to generate new brain cells decreases, we may start feeling low, become depressed, and exhibit poorer memory; in contrast, we know that being active can double the regeneration rate of brain cells—it truly has that much of an impact.

136

Move more and develop a more nuanced worldview

The hippocampus, our memory center, is made up of several parts. Neurogenesis happens primarily in one of these parts—the *gyrus dentatus*—the dentate gyrus. It's interesting that the production of brain cells happens right in that spot. The dentate gyrus has a very specific function that is important for what is called *pattern separation*, the ability to register small, subtle differences in what is happening around you, compared to earlier events. Let's say you enter a room where a cocktail party is in full swing. One of the guests is your sister, a few are close friends of yours, and a few others are casual acquaintances that you have only met a few times. There are also some people you've never met before.

When you see your sister, you recognize her immediately. Your brain doesn't have to work very hard to identify her. Same goes with your friends. However, when you see people whom you've only met once or twice, your brain begins matching their faces to what is in your memory bank. "*Who* is that? I know her so well. She looks like someone from my old job, but no—that's not her, because she was taller and had lighter hair."

When you must think so hard that it hurts to try and remember who is in front of you, your dentate gyrus is in overdrive trying to match the face with memories of people you've met before. By sifting through minute differences in, say, hair color, height, or facial features, the dentate gyrus is trying to decide if you know this person. He or she can remind you of someone else, and it is by noticing the little details that you'll figure out if this is someone you have met before or if he or she is completely unknown to you.

Much of what we experience resembles things we have already lived. Think back at what you've done today. How many activities were truly unique, things you've never done before? Probably not much is distinct, unless you live a very varied life.

Even though many things remind us of stuff we've done before and many people we meet remind us of others we've crossed paths with, it's up to our brain to store information on similar events and people as separate memories that can be told apart. That's what pattern separation is: the crucial ability to have a nuanced view of our environment. Without it, our memories would just flit together into a fog and render us incapable of telling one from the other. Consequently, the regeneration of cells happens right in the part of the brain that is important for pattern separation. You can assertively claim—especially if you are physically active—that exercising improves the odds of having a more nuanced worldview. Personally, I believe that this could be why physical activity is so effective in treating depression.

A person suffering from depression leads a reduced emotional life and ends up missing life's little subtleties—he or she feels that things are gray and dreary. On the other hand, the opportunities of catching a more nuanced glance at life—and glimmers of hope—may just increase thanks to the regeneration of brain cells in the dentate gyrus.

Does only exercise count?

Does only exercise count in increasing the regeneration of brain cells? Can more stimulating surroundings—what scientists call an *enriched environment*—also be important for the brain's ability to create new cells? Yes, environment also plays a role. How many new cells we make doesn't only depend on how many cells are created, but also on how many of those cells we get to keep. New brain cells are incredibly fragile, and only one in two cells survives. However, it looks like it's possible to raise the odds of survival so that more of them can make it. In animals living in a more enriched environment, about 80 percent of new brain cells remain viable.

Exercise and physical activity favors the production of additional brain cells, and a stimulating environment increases the odds that those cells will survive. It's totally logical that these two are linked: we have evolved to experience new environments and events as we move about, and the brain is prepared to take in new information. To increase our ability to remember what we experience, new cells are created in the hippocampus. Then, what we experience as we move around in this new environment provides the stimulation that ensures the survival of these cells.

138

We can conclude that exercise and physical training lay the groundwork for the brain to learn new things. Is it now beginning to seem less strange that we can recall up to 20 percent more words if we walk while we listen to them? I thought so.

Our inbuilt emotional brake and GPS

While the hippocampus helps us build long-term memories, its responsibilities don't end there. The hippocampus is also important for its ability to help us put things into perspective and compare what we're experiencing presently with other memories so we don't overreact emotionally. Furthermore, it plays an important role in our ability to place ourselves spatially, like a brain GPS that keeps track of our position and allows us to store memories of places (a discovery that was awarded the Nobel Prize in Medicine in 2014, by the way). As we read this, specific cells in the hippocampus signal where we are inside, or outside, the room. If we move by a few inches, other hippocampus cells that function as "place cells" become active and create an inner map of our surroundings.

In other words, the hippocampus has a list of important functions other than being a memory center, such as controlling our emotions, keeping track of us spatially, and making sure we can find our way around locations we've been in before. The more we learn about the hippocampus, the more we realize the importance of this part of the brain. If the hippocampus doesn't work, neither does the brain.

There is a reason why I've devoted so many pages to describing the hippocampus: it's the part of the brain that is perhaps most influenced by us moving our bodies. We've learned that physical activity leads to the birth of new cells in the hippocampus. The hippocampus gets more energy when blood flow increases, allowing it to function better. Also, the existing hippocampus cells seem to become genetically younger, and the shrinking that occurs with aging can be slowed down, perhaps even turned around. Over the long haul, the hippocampus—and therefore the whole brain—works better and more effectively in people who exercise regularly.

139

Those of you who train will notice that the hippocampus is strengthened in several different ways. Aside from your memory improving, you will eventually realize that you're not as emotional as before and don't react as strongly to negative events. It might also affect how well you find your way around different places. Moreover, many who train find that they make quicker and better associations—in other words, they think quicker on their feet—which could be due to a strong hippocampus.

Different types of exercise affect different kinds of memory

Even if memories are spread out all over the brain, different areas specialize in handling different kinds of memories. The frontal lobe and the hippocampus are important for working memory, as in being able to keep a phone number in your head while you dial it. The hippocampus is also important for remembering places.

The temporal lobe is key to *episodic memory*, which is how you remember, say, what happened on Christmas Eve. To a great extent, memories are stored in the same area as they are used, so visual memories are stored primarily in the visual cortex.

Fascinatingly, it seems that different types of movement can influence the brain's different areas in a variety of ways. This leads us to wonder if different types of training have an impact on different kinds of memories. For example, it has been shown that word recall is boosted by running, but not by lifting weights. However, weight training appears to be good for *associative memory*, which is the ability to pair a name with a face. When it comes to remembering where you put the keys, both running and weight training seem to do the trick.

We can draw two conclusions from studying these effects more closely. First, and most important, if you wish to strengthen your memory, you must be physically active in some way or another. What you choose to do is not important. Second, if you want to boost all your memory areas, from remembering where you've set stuff down to the words you've read, you should vary your training and make sure to do cardiovascular

140

Regular exercise might even influence how quickly you think on your feet.

exercise and weight training. However, if you must choose between the two, cardio should take priority, since it is more beneficial for memory.

That both the hippocampus and the frontal lobe are strengthened by exercise means that physical activity should be able to improve many areas of your memory, and it's possible that both short-term memory (where you remember stuff for a few minutes or hours) and long-term memory improve. Even if most research has focused on the effects of exercise on short-term memory, physical activity should boost all memory, whether it concerns what happened this morning or something that took place twenty years ago!

WHAT ELSE IS INVOLVED IN THE REGENERATION OF NEW BRAIN CELLS?

Besides exercise, things like sex, a low-calorie diet (but not starvation), and flavonoids found in, say, plain chocolate are all associated with an increase in the neurogenesis rate of new brain cells. A decrease in new cells can be caused by stress, lack of sleep, too much alcohol, and a high-fat diet, especially one high in saturated fat found in butter and cheese.

PHYSICAL TRAINING VS. COMPUTER GAMES

If you Google the term *cognitive training,* you'll get more than ten million results. Most are ads for apps, games, and other products that purport to make your brain more effective. It is certainly a tempting offer, because who doesn't want to have a better-functioning brain? Training the brain via different methods has, in a very short time, become a multibillion industry; every year more than ten billion dollars in cognitive training games are sold.

Recently, seventy of the world's most eminent neuroscientists and psychologists, under the auspices of Stanford University and the Max Planck Institute, decided to see whether there was any merit to these game and app manufacturers' claims. The experts scoured the scientific studies on cognitive training to find answers to the question of whether games improved cognitive abilities.

Their conclusion came back in the form of scathing criticism. It was found that cognitive training methods proffered by games and apps do not make you smarter, more focused, or more creative, and you do not improve your memory. You simply get better at playing the game. The same conclusion was found with crosswords and Sudoku, which are often referred to as brain gymnastics. If you work at filling in crosswords, you'll get better at completing crosswords, but not at anything else.

By contrast, research has shown time and again that exercise and physical activity can truly strengthen all our cognitive functions. If you're still on the fence about this, it just means that you haven't read this book properly! In the race between physical and cognitive exercises, physical exercise wins by a mile.

142

THE RIGHT PRESCRIPTION FOR IMPROVED MEMORY

Ideally, you should alternate between cardiovascular (endurance) exercise and weight training. Most of the research has focused on aerobic training's effect on the hippocampus, but it looks like some effects on memory can only, or at least mostly, be achieved by training with weights.

Train before or while learning something.

Don't go all-out—a walk or a light jog is all that's required.

Train regularly. Of course, you can improve your memory with a single workout, but just like the effects on many of our cognitive faculties, our memory improves much more if you're patient and keep up your training over several continuous months.

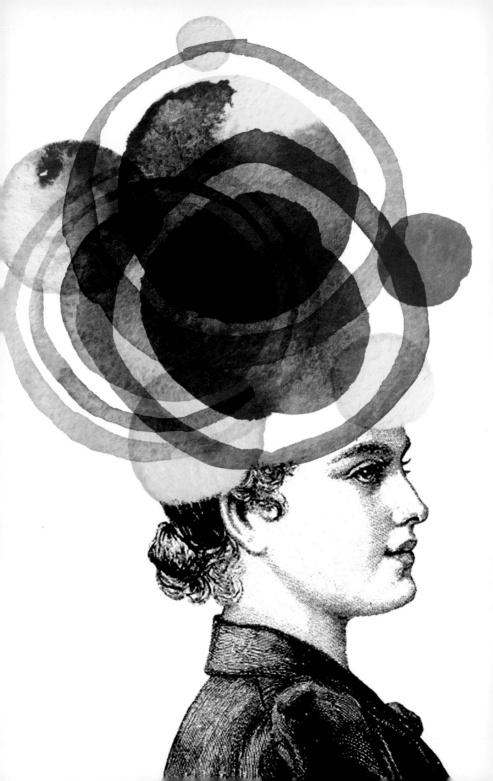

6. TRAIN YOURSELF TO BE CREATIVE

*The moment my legs begin to move
my thoughts begin to flow.*
HENRY DAVID THOREAU

The widely-known Japanese author Haruki Murakami has books that have sold millions of copies around the world. He can line up his many prestigious literary awards in a long row, and his name is regularly put forward for the Nobel Prize in Literature. Anyone who wonders where Murakami gets his inspiration need not look further than the title of his 2008 autobiography, *What I Talk About When I Talk About Running*. In the book, Murakami describes his creative process in detail: When he is writing, he gets up at 4 a.m. and works until 10 a.m.; then he goes for a ten-kilometer run after lunch and follows that up with a swim. He spends the rest of the day listening to music and reading. He goes to bed around 9 p.m. He follows this routine seven days a week for six months, until the book he is working on is finished. To get things done, Murakami needs the physical strength he gets from training, which he considers as essential to the writing process as his creativity.

Murakami is far from alone in having discovered the immeasurable effects exercise can have on one's creative energy. There is a slew of authors, musicians, actors, artists, scientists, and entrepreneurs who have borne witness to how they use exercise to become more creative.

TRAIN YOURSELF TO BE CREATIVE

IDEAS JUST TUMBLED OUT AFTER A RUN

Exercise's effects on creativity was one of the reasons I became interested in how the brain is influenced by physical activity. I often had good ideas after I'd been out for a run or after a game of tennis. At first I thought it was just a fluke, or perhaps I had simply become more alert. But it happened time and time again, and the effect was so tangible in the hours after my exercise that I began to wonder if the workouts were actually making me more creative. When I found out about the studies on creativity and physical activity, it became clear that what I was experiencing wasn't just because I felt happier and more alert.

Boost your creativity with a walk

Many highly creative people have testified to how exercise has worked wonders for their creativity. It is said that Albert Einstein discovered the theory of relativity while on a bike ride. Beethoven, one of the greatest musical geniuses who has ever lived, composed three symphonies despite going deaf in his forties. He often took a break during the day, during which he went on long walks for inspiration. Charles Darwin took hour-long strolls around his home at Down House—on a loop he called his "thinking path." It was during a period of extended rambles that Darwin developed his groundbreaking work on the origin of species, perhaps the most important work ever in the field of biology.

A more current example is Apple's late cofounder and CEO Steve Jobs, who held regular walking meetings because he felt they were more productive than meetings that took place around a conference room table. He seems to have inspired many of Silicon Valley's elite, such as Facebook founder Mark Zuckerberg and Twitter's Jack Dorsey, to do the same.

DIFFERENT TYPES OF CREATIVITY

While these anecdotes on exercise's beneficial influence on creativity are revealing, they're lacking in hard evidence. Before we can claim that physical activity can get you to think outside the box—and how you can best achieve this—we need to find out what creativity is, and how you test for it.

For anything to be deemed creative, it needs to be both new and meaningful. Copying someone else's work isn't particularly creative. Besides, what is created must fulfill some purpose or function, because a pointless invention isn't very creative, either.

In the study of innovation, a distinction is often made between two kinds of creativity: divergent and convergent thinking. Divergent thinking is the classic brainstorming: coming up with many different solutions to a problem by thinking broadly and using plenty of associations. A typical test for divergent thinking is called the *Alternative Uses Test*, which is based on word association. For example, you're given a word like *brick,* and, while being timed, you must come up with as many uses as you can for a brick—to build a wall in a house, to use as a paperweight or a doorstop. It isn't just the number of answers that is important, but also how detailed those answers are and how different they are from one another. Preferably, the answers should be unique and not repeat what other test subjects have already mentioned. However, completely unrealistic answers, like using the brick to build a space rocket, don't count.

This test might sound simplistic, but it has been shown to reflect a person's level of creativity very accurately; and I can attest to the fact that this experiment is not simple, especially when time is monitored. The big advantage of this test is that it measures creativity only, and not IQ; people with high IQs don't do better than others. In fact, they often get stuck when they do this test.

Convergent thinking is almost diametrically opposite to divergent thinking. Here, it's not a matter of brainstorming a variety of solutions, but of quickly arriving at one answer—the correct one—which often boils down to a common denominator. An example would be that you are given three words, and you must quickly find what they have in common. Let's say the words are *Central Park*, the *Museum of Modern Art*, and the *Empire State Building*—what all these have in common is that they are tourist attractions in New York City. In other words, there is just one correct answer, or a few; the rest of the answers are wrong. Convergent thinking emphasizes speed and logic more than divergent thinking and is more taxing on the brain. Nevertheless, convergent thinking is important for creativity, in artistic as well as scientific endeavors.

Give your ideas some legs

Lately, thanks to these tests, we have scientific proof that physical activity boosts creativity. One of the more elegant studies on the topic was conducted by scientists at Stanford University, in which they asked 176 subjects to perform several different creativity tests. Some performed the tests after having walked, and others did them after resting.

The study's title "Give your ideas some legs: the positive effect of walking on creative thinking" provides a clue as to the outcome. Over four out of five test subjects performed better on the tests when they did them while moving about. The differences weren't insignificant, either. On average, the test results of those who walked while being tested were 60 percent better than those who had not walked, primarily in their ability to brainstorm and generate new ideas. However, convergent thinking (i.e., the ability to find the right answer and/or a common denominator) did not improve. This basically illustrates that physical activity seems to boost idea generation rather than logic. The coauthor of the study, Marily Oppezzo, made the following statement: "We do not proclaim that walks will turn you into a modern-day Michelangelo, but they can help you to get going in the initial stages of the creative process."

Movement is more important than environment and temperament

A shift in one's surroundings is said to stimulate a different way of thinking. There could be some truth to this, of course, but the Stanford

> *Walks might not turn you into a modern-day Michelangelo, but they can help you to get going in the initial stages of the creative process.*

study showed that it didn't matter where the walk took place for creativity to improve. Some test subjects walked outside around the university campus while others walked inside on a treadmill, where they only had a gray wall to stare at. Despite this, creativity was improved in both those who walked outside and those who walked on the treadmill.

To make sure it was the walking that impacting the creative thinking and not the environment, some of the test subjects were pushed around in wheelchairs on the campus walking path. In other words, they were in the same surroundings as those who had walked outside but were not physically active. The result? It was not the environment that affected creativity, because creativity increased much more in the group that had walked on the path compared to the group that had been wheeled along that same path. A change of environment did not appear to have any effect on creativity. What matters is that we walk or run, not where we do it.

What about temper? Since our mood improves after physical activity, increased creativity could be explained by the fact that those who had trained felt better overall. However, that doesn't seem to be the case. Creativity tests that were performed after exercise have shown that even the subjects who did not feel better after the training still performed better on the tests after training.

Thus, improved creativity is not the result of just feeling better. In other words, getting fresh ideas is linked to physical activity and cannot be explained by extenuating circumstances such as a change of environment or mood.

150

Should you run or walk?

The test subjects of the Stanford University study walked around the campus, but what is optimal for increasing creativity—should you walk or run? Even if it isn't entirely possible to say for sure, it seems one could postulate that running, or moving in an equally vigorous way, is better than walking. Making a little more of an effort does indeed seem to pay off, but you need to keep it up for at least thirty minutes. Improved creativity expresses itself mainly *after* exercise, which is obviously an ideal situation. You can brainstorm while walking, but not so much while running.

How long do we remain creative after moving around? Does it last for the rest of our life? Sadly, no. The creative boost is quite short-lived; it increases anywhere from one to a few hours after exertion, and then it wears off. If we want another jolt of inspiration, we must go for another walk or run, just like Haruki Murakami and his daily runs. However, from a creative standpoint, it is unwise to go all-out to the point of exhaustion, because that will not improve creativity—experiments have demonstrated that people who push too hard tend to perform worse on creativity tests after their workouts.

We do not know why the benefits are so short-lived and why they disappear if we become too fatigued. We know that blood flow to the brain increases when we move around. When the brain gets more blood, it works more efficiently, and cognitive abilities—among them, creativity—improve. However, if we work out to the point of exhaustion, blood flow to the brain decreases instead since blood is now redirected from the brain to the muscles, where it is needed to provide us with maximum performance. Less blood in the brain seems to lead to lesser mental capabilities.

Perhaps there have been times where you've had a hard time thinking clearly when you've been exhausted? Be that as it may, it's important to emphasize that the dip in creativity that follows fatigue is only temporary; nothing suggests that creativity dwindles over the long term due to hard training.

Make sure to start out fit

Does everyone who trains become more creative, or is there a catch? Yes, there is, and it's that you need to be reasonably fit to see good results. Fit people actually perform better on creativity tests if they are done in tandem with physical activity. Creativity doesn't seem to improve at all in people who are not fit; in fact, it seems that it worsens a few hours after training, at least if the training session appears to be intense. This is probably from the decrease in blood flow to the brain due to exhaustion; even a short run at an unhurried pace can be exhausting for an unfit individual.

So, if you want to boost your creativity by exercising, you need to make sure you're in reasonably good shape to see a positive outcome. If you're not at that point yet but still wish to strengthen your creativity by training, it's best to walk or jog at a leisurely pace so you don't drain your tanks completely.

Ingenuity or hard work?

In a preserved letter, Mozart explains how he composes his music. The process seems completely magical. The legendary composer describes how he creates musical masterpieces without even going near an instrument: he hears complete pieces in his head, and then he quite simply writes them down on paper, as if they had already been composed. Later, when it is performed by a symphony orchestra, the music sounds as wonderful as when he first heard it in his head.

This image of an artistic genius's enormous creative powers is undoubtedly very compelling, and it's often used to illustrate how the brains of extremely creative people work in ways that we mere mortals can scarcely imagine. Problem is, that letter is a fake. Mozart didn't compose his symphonies that way at all. Everything suggests that he worked with determination, and that he used music theory as well as other established methods to write. He spent endless hours fine-tuning his pieces, reworking, modifying, and reworking them again until he was satisfied. Mozart's classical masterpieces are more the product of hard work than of some whimsical effort.

A similar story involves Newton and how he arrived at his theory about gravity—just like that, when an apple fell on his head while he was sitting under a tree. What is not recounted, however, are the decades he toiled in mathematics and physics before the idea struck him. It then took him twenty years from the apple incident for Newton's complete theory to be fully articulated.

Of course, Mozart and Newton might have had their "Eureka!" moments, but everything indicates that their flashes of brilliance didn't hit them haphazardly and were instead products of a long and painstaking slog. This doesn't mean that everyone who makes the effort can compose timeless music like Mozart or make trailblazing contributions to science like Newton, but it certainly means that we can all practice and fine-tune our creative abilities if we try.

Quantity leads to quality

Do you belong to that category of people who come up with plenty of concepts; make free-associations right, left, and center; and suggest one thing after another when brainstorming? Or do you belong to those who only suggest a few things and hope they'll be good enough? It's a fact that the first process has proven to be the best way to come up with the most ideas.

When we study how people perform on creativity tests for divergent thinking, those who have lots of ideas also tend to have a greater number of *good* ideas. This may sound obvious, but it's worth looking closer at the implications. If you generate a lot of ideas, chances are likelier that you will hit upon a good one, even if the rest are bad. It's not as common to come up with only one or two ideas that are brilliant, with no throwaways.

For most of us to think up ideas, we must put in more effort. That importance of perseverance in creativity is underrated, as evidenced by the fictional tales of Mozart and Newton. Exercise isn't just beneficial for divergent and convergent thinking; it also helps to give us the energy to keep plugging away with ideas. When you become physically and mentally stronger through physical activity, your stamina for additional work increases—as exemplified by Haruki Murakami during his intense bouts of writing—and so the good ideas tend to pop up sooner or later.

HOW CREATIVITY WORKS

Our knowledge about what happens in the brain when we're being creative has advanced by leaps and bounds; we no longer consider the creative process some sort of black box that we don't know how to operate.

We have begun to understand *why* some people are more creative than others. Researchers on creativity have not only directed their interest toward the areas of the brain like the frontal lobe (the seat of our higher cognitive functions); the trail also seems to lead to an area deeper inside the brain: the *thalamus*.

The thalamus sorts out information

An enormous amount of information is constantly being triaged inside our brain: what we're seeing and hearing at this very moment; how our arms and legs are positioned; if it's warm or cold in the room; how often our lungs fill with air as we breathe; and how quickly our heart beats. Our brain receives this information continuously, day and night. We're conscious of some of these data, and unaware of the rest. We typically don't give much thought to our breathing or how our legs are placed, and it must be so for us to function normally. If all this information reached our consciousness, we wouldn't be able to concentrate on anything besides our initial impressions.

The thalamus refers to the part of the brain that acts as a kind of filter for our consciousness to prevent us from becoming overwhelmed by information. The thalamus is situated in the brain like the hub of a bicycle wheel where all the spokes meet; it's not by accident that the location of the thalamus is so central. Information is gathered in the thalamus from the brain's different areas (like the centers for visual impressions, for example), at which point it chooses which signals are let through to our consciousness. The thalamus is like an executive assistant who picks which meetings her boss—in this case, the cerebral cortex and our consciousness—should attend, and which ones he can sit out. If the thalamus doesn't function properly, the cerebral cortex runs the risk of becoming overloaded with information and not working as it should— like a secretary who is unable to make decisions and who arranges meetings all over the place, causing her boss, who is in meetings all the time, to work inefficiently.

To think outside the box

Today, we believe that this kind of information overload is what happens in the psychiatric disorder we call *schizophrenia*, where the sufferer loses touch with reality and experiences symptoms such as delusions and hallucinations. Many things point to the schizophrenic's brain receiving too many strong impressions at once, making it hard for him or her to hang on to the real world. This leads the afflicted individual to subconsciously create an alternative picture of his or her surroundings. Schizophrenics often exhibit very bizarre thought patterns. Occasionally, I have met some who cling to such weird delusions that I could never have made up myself along those same lines, no matter how hard I tried.

But there are always two sides to a coin. Having a thalamus that lets through a lot of information isn't always a weakness or something that leads to mental illness. It also appears to be related to creativity; it can lead us to make unsuspected associations and think outside the box. If our cerebral cortex and consciousness receive many signals, it increases our chances of having unique ideas and seeing things from a different perspective.

So how does our brain work? For the thalamus filter to function normally, we need dopamine (yes, it plays an important role here, too), but not too much of it and not too little—just enough. If dopamine levels deviate from the correct amount, the thalamus might not let the right number of signals through, leading to information overload, which can either be a benefit or a drawback.

In other words, various dopamine levels in the thalamus could be linked to increased creativity *and* mental illness. This in fact appears to be the case. We know from experiments performed by Swedish professor and neuroscientist Fredrik Ullén at the Swedish Karolinska Institute that people who perform especially well on creativity tests for divergent thinking have fewer dopamine receivers in the thalamus, causing them to register unusual levels of dopamine. Consequently, their thalamus lets through more signals, and their thinking is more creative.

What's interesting is that the same thing has been observed in schizophrenics who perform well on creativity tests—they seem to have fewer dopamine receptors in the thalamus—but for them, this leads to psychosis instead of creative thinking. So what decides whether we'll become mentally ill or creative geniuses? We don't know for sure right now. Perhaps if our brain already works well in other ways, the increased flow of information can become an asset instead of a liability; it could be that the brain is resilient enough to handle the strain of added data without having to resort to creating alternative realities. You are original and creative and can free-associate in unusual ways without becoming psychotic. However, if your brain can't process things normally, it won't be able to handle the deluge of information, and so you could suffer from psychosis and lose touch with reality.

When it comes to the brain, things are seldom in black and white, where you either possess an ability or you don't. It isn't that people who let a large load of information go through the thalamus are either creative or psychotic. There are gray zones in which you can show signs of qualities, but to different extents. There is a vast spectrum between creativity and mental illness along which people are situated. Some may have to deal with a lot of data, and their brain is hanging on for dear life to cope with the load. At certain times in their lives, they may show symptoms bordering on psychosis, while at other times, when their brain is running smoothly, they can create things that others can only dream about.

A hairline fissure separates madness from genius

There are lots of people throughout history who have shown us how close creativity is to madness. Two famous cases are the artist Vincent van Gogh and the philosopher Friedrich Nietzsche, who were both enormously creative, yet who also suffered from mental illness at different times of their lives. A later example is John Nash, a Nobel Prize winner in economics, who combined exceptional creativity with serious mental problems. Nash, portrayed by Russell Crowe in the Oscar-winning movie *A Beautiful Mind*, was one of the world's leading mathematicians who also happened to suffer from schizophrenia. He heard voices and was delusional, believing that he was being followed, threatened, and conspired against. He found his affliction to be both a blessing and a curse. "I would never have had such good scientific ideas had I been able to think normally," he said about his exceptional creative abilities.

Many highly creative people don't suffer from mental illness, but they can trace it in their family. One of the greatest minds of our age, Albert Einstein, had a son who was schizophrenic. Polymath Bertrand Russell, who was a philosopher, an author, and a politician, had many relatives who suffered from schizophrenia. David Bowie, one of the past decades' musical luminaries, had a schizophrenic brother.

One possible explanation for this link is that both the creative people and their disabled relatives had a bigger rush of information through the thalamus—a more intense thought flow—but some of them had a brain that could handle the excess data and knew how to make use of it. This is what made them geniuses. Meanwhile, their relatives, who had brains that weren't as resilient, became mentally ill.

157

Boost the flow of ideas, and your ability to handle them

The frontal lobe is seemingly vital for us to channel the flow of ideas through the thalamus and make something out of them. As we've already seen, training strengthens the frontal lobe. It does it in the short term by increasing blood flow, causing the frontal lobe to work better, and over the long term through other mechanisms we will read more about in the chapter *Improved concentration*. Exercise and training improves the conditions for using our flow of ideas and turning them into something productive.

Additionally, exercise doesn't merely affect our ability to handle the flow of ideas; it is also likely to influence the actual flow of ideas. We're not sure exactly what kind of mechanisms are responsible for this, but one possibility is that physical activity affects dopamine, which is critical to the filter in the thalamus. However, with dopamine it's not always the case that more—or less—is always better. The systems in the brain are incredibly complex, and theories of too much or too little of one thing or the other are often far too simplistic. Instead, one way to see this is that the different systems are more or less in tune, and exercise fine-tunes the dopamine system, influencing how you feel and how much information the thalamus lets through, thereby affecting how creative you are.

We're born with an individual range of basic creative talent, and we can't change that. What we do with that talent later is, however, up to us. There are many different factors that are important for creativity, but the fact is that physical activity is one of the most important. Are you stuck on a problem at work? Are you having trouble finding a good idea for a book you'd like to write or a company you want to launch? If so, get out there and run! If it can work wonders for Haruki Murakami and for Beethoven, it should also be able to help you and me.

TRAIN YOURSELF TO BE CREATIVE

THE RIGHT PRESCRIPTION TO INCREASE CREATIVITY

The best way to boost creativity is to go for a run or to be active in a similarly vigorous way. A walk is good, too, but it won't be as effective.

Run for at least twenty to thirty minutes. You'll feel the effect on your creativity afterward, and it will last for about two hours.

Don't run to the point of exhaustion, because creativity diminishes for several hours after a hard workout (not over the long term, though).

Make sure that you're fit, because that is when the effect of exercise on creativity is the strongest.

Training improves the ability to brainstorm, primarily, but that might differ from person to person.

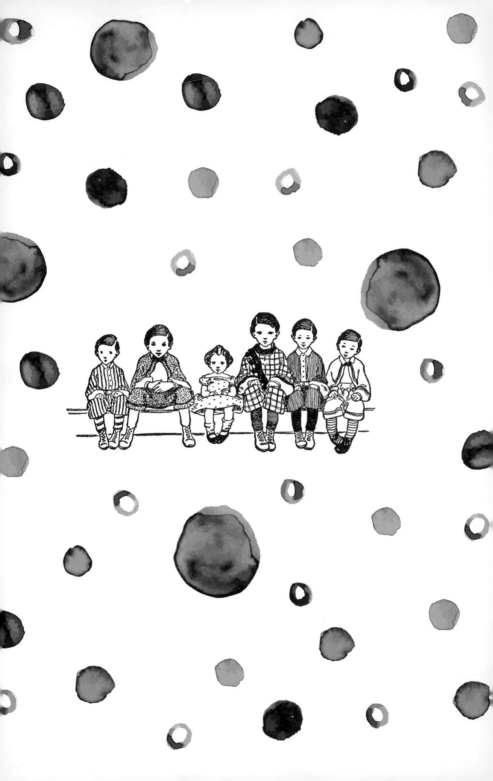

7. THE GROWING BRAIN

For children to reach their full potential,
they need to be active.
CATHERINE DAVIS

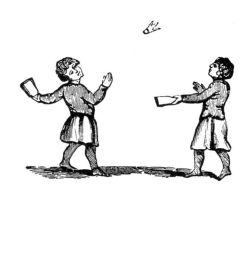

The Program for International Student Assessment test (PISA) measures the scholastic performance of fifteen-year-olds and is used to compare the academic prowess of students across different countries. In December of 2013, the latest results of the PISA test were presented, and they were a bombshell to my native Sweden. Swedish students weren't merely light-years behind countries such as South Korea, Singapore, and Hong Kong, which topped the list. They also performed worse than average compared to other OECD (The Organization for Economic Cooperation and Development) countries and came in last among our Nordic neighbors. Math, reading, and scientific levels were in an especially sorry state. Worst of all, we were heading in the wrong direction—Sweden was the country whose rankings had fallen the farthest.

Lively debates have since ensued, and many appear to have ideas on how to turn this situation around. But maybe the discussion should center less on teaching methods and class size and focus more on what research has shown to have a formidable influence on children's memory and learning abilities—that they be physically active. Today, children simply do not get enough physical education.

It's certainly not only what happens in class that affects a child's instruction; research has clearly shown that movement has a reinforcing effect on children's and teenagers' ability to learn. School athletics are about so much more than what takes place on the soccer field or in the gymnasium—it's definitely not about winning teams or making children good at certain sports. School athletics is about improving the groundwork for learning math and English.

MORE GYM CLASSES—HIGHER MATH GRADES

The most convincing proof that exercise improves children's academic results in the "three Rs" (reading, writing, and arithmetic) doesn't come from some American Ivy League university, but from Bunkeflo, a suburb in the Swedish southern region of Skåne. There, two elementary school classes were followed as they participated in athletics every day. Another elementary class at the same school was used as a control group, and they engaged in the customary two gym classes per week.

The groups of kids were comparable in every respect, other than the amount of sports they took part in. They all lived in the same area, attended the same school, and studied the same subjects. What happened next? For starters, those who went to gym every day got better grades in gym class than the others—no surprise there. What was unexpected, however, was that they also did better in math, Swedish, and English without receiving any extra tutoring in these subjects. And the effects continued over many years; more of the kids who had extra gym classes graduated from the ninth grade with satisfactory grades than those in the control group. The effect was especially noticeable among the boys. Typically, girls get better grades than boys, but the grades leveled out completely between the genders of the children who participated in a daily gym class. No other approach has provided this kind of outcome.

It's not only in Skåne that we've seen this link. American scientists also noticed it when they studied some 250 elementary school children in third and fifth grades. A measuring technique was used that took cardiovascular fitness, muscle strength, and agility into consideration to paint a complete picture of the participants' physical fitness. They also looked at how well the children did academically. Here too, the results were unambiguous: physically fit children did better at math and reading comprehension. The higher their fitness levels, the higher their grades. The opposite was true for overweight children: the more overweight the kid was, the worse his or her test scores were. The widely-held preconceived notion that overweight children are academically minded and physically active children are empty-headed has proven to be completely baseless.

Is it risky to draw conclusions from a study of only 250 children or of a few elementary school classes in Skåne? In Nebraska, nearly twelve thousand children were tested, and results indicated that the fitter children tested better in math and English than those who were unfit. However, excess weight—a major concern in the US—didn't play a role in the findings. Overweight children scored neither better not worse than the children of normal weight.

So how can exercise make children better at math and languages? As you've read in the chapter *Jog your memory*, physical activity makes the hippocampus—our center for memory and emotional control—grow in adults who are physically active. This appears to happen in children, too.

When the brains of ten-year-olds were examined by MRI, it showed that fit children had bigger hippocampi, one of the most important areas of the brain. These variations even went hand in hand with the finding that fit children did better on memory tests. So, good physical fitness leads to a larger hippocampus *and* better results on memory tests.

What's more, the more complex the tests, the bigger the difference between the fit and unfit children. On simple memory tests, the variance isn't too distinct; it's on the difficult tests that the fit children do much better.

One single training session produces results

Just as exercise has an immediate impact on the adult brain, the same quick, strengthening benefit takes effect in children's brains. When nine-year-olds were physically active for twenty minutes—in one single session—they became markedly better at reading. One short burst of

When nine-year-olds were physically active for one twenty-minute session, they improved markedly on their reading comprehension. One short burst of activity affected the kids' academic abilities!

exercise altered the kids' academic abilities! Why this happens we don't know for sure, but we are certain that children's attention spans improve immediately after they are physically active; as a result, we can assume that attention span has an important role to play in this context.

In the same way that we've examined the *minimum* amount of training required for adults to see an improvement in fitness, we've checked to see how *little* training is needed to improve the attention span of children. The results are astonishing! When teenagers jogged for twelve minutes, both their reading comprehension and what is called *visual attention* improved. The effect lasted the better part of an hour, but a bout of activity as brief as four minutes (yes, you read that right!) can improve our ability to stay focused and alert and can get ten-year-olds to remain undistracted.

Attention span and memory are not the only things that improve in children who are physically active. Today we know that physically active kids between the ages of four and eighteen will show improvement in practically *all* of their cognitive faculties. Multitasking, working memory, and focus—everything seems to get better. The same goes for the ability to make decisions (i.e., executive control).

Executive control might sound like a trait only company directors need to have. However, even children need to be able to show initiative and make decisions. They need to be able to plan, to organize, and to stay focused on what they are doing in the present, even when they're distracted by, say, their cell phones. Children must also be able to stop themselves from giving in to every single impulse they feel. Thus, it's not exactly rash to say that executive control is necessary for children to do well academically.

Less stressed children

It's true that the effects of being physically active in childhood have positive results that go far beyond academic success and proper executive control. Kids also become less sensitive to stress. Two hundred and fifty-eight Finnish second-graders were studied to see how they reacted to stressful situations, and whether there was a connection between their vulnerability to stress and their level of physical activity. Asking nine-year-olds how active they are does not yield reliable answers, so the kids were outfitted with pedometers. Their stress resilience was measured by administering tests that mimicked daily stressors, such as being timed while doing arithmetic or giving presentations to one another—situations that are deemed just as high-stress for children as for adults.

Turns out, the connection was obvious. Children who took a lot of steps every day didn't react as strongly to stress as the kids who didn't walk as much. And it didn't just show in their calmer demeanor: the levels of the stress hormone cortisol didn't rise as much in the physically active children as in the sedentary kids when they completed high-stress arithmetic and presentation tests. If anything, this is strong evidence that physically active children are more resilient to stress.

I completely understand how easy it is to feel guilty when reading about these studies, especially if you have children who aren't interested in gym or sports and who are glued to their computers. How do you go about making them active? A good starting point is to let your kid pick what he or she enjoys doing. American scientists tried this tactic by letting overweight elementary school children, who were not into gym

166

activities and who were mostly sedentary in their free time, get together and be physically active during after-school hours. To get the children to join in, they let them choose an activity they thought would be fun, so long as they did something. Some kids ran, some jumped rope, and some played ball sports. The outcome was that the kids improved in math without having to take extra lessons. The more physically active they became, the more their math scores improved, even though they hadn't completed any extra class work. Twenty short minutes of exercise produced results, but the kids who saw the most improvement were active for at least forty minutes and had increased their heart rate substantially, preferably up to 150 beats per minute.

But these positive effects didn't stop at improved math comprehension. A few of the overweight kids who did not like sports and who had been encouraged to become active were examined by MRI. The images showed that the activity in the prefrontal cortex—the area behind the forehead and our center for abstract thinking, concentration, and planning—had risen. The study's authors summarized this finding in a way that numbers or tables could not come close to doing: "For children to reach their full potential, they need to be active."

In the short term and long term

When we fit the pieces of the puzzle together, the amazing effect that exercise has on children's brains becomes obvious, both in the short term and long term. A single bout of activity increases attention span and improves concentration and reading comprehension. It continues to do so for one to several hours, before it wears off. Like adults, children reap significant, long-term benefits if they exercise regularly for several months. Again, as with adults, the choice of activity is not of much import. Running, playing, competing in tennis or soccer—all seem to have the same positive impact. What is vital is raising the heart rate. The critical thing is not what the children do to be physically active; it's that they *are* physically active.

167

From the brain development's perspective, is there an age at which we should be especially mindful that our kids exercise? We don't know that in detail yet, but many clues suggest that children of elementary school age reap the most benefits from being active.

Exercise strengthens different areas in the child's brain

We know how physical activity strengthens the adult brain; we also know that a child's brain changes with physical activity. Furthermore, we know what happens inside the brain. We can tease the brain into gray and white matter. The gray matter, also called the *cerebral cortex*, is the brain's outermost layer. It measures a few millimeters in thickness, and it isn't gray but rather more of a shade of pink due to all the blood vessels that provide the brain with blood. It's in the gray matter that sophisticated activity takes place. Information is sorted and memories are stored. One can deduce that this is where the "magic" happens because of all the energy it consumes. Gray matter uses over 90 percent of the brain's total energy needs, even though it makes up about 40 percent of the brain's volume.

The white matter lies beneath the gray matter, and it passes information along between the different areas of the brain. It's made up of long projections (called *axons*) from the nerve cells, which brain cells use to communicate with one another. Imagine the gray matter as a bunch of computers, and the white matter as cables that pass signals between the computers.

The pale coloring of the white matter is from the axons being insulated with a substance called *myelin*, which contains a lot of fat. Myelin improves the signal reception between the brain cells.

Both the gray and the white matter are vital to how we function. The gray matter does indeed perform most of the heavy lifting, but if the axons aren't effective and can't transmit the signals, the brain won't work properly. That makes sense; a computer can only run if all its parts are properly connected.

168

What changes most in children who are physically active, the gray or the white matter? Both! Growth of gray matter is first noticed in the hippocampus (which is part of the gray matter); however, white matter is also strengthened by exercise and training. Children who are physically active regularly show alteration in white matter. Like gray matter, it becomes thicker and more compact. This almost certainly means that it's becoming more efficient. In science, we call this *white matter integrity*.

To bring back the metaphor of white matter acting as cables between computers, it appears that the connection works better in physically active children. This means that information is transmitted more efficiently between the different areas of the brain, making the entire brain run better.

There's no doubt that gray matter is essential to cognitive ability, but it looks like the same goes for white matter, too. In fact, white matter has been specifically linked to academic performance. When elementary school children's brains were examined by DTI (Diffusion Tensor Imaging)—an extremely advanced medical technique—the scans showed that white matter in the left side of the brain is related to mathematical ability. We can't say for sure if it's the strengthening of white matter that's responsible for making fit children do better in school, but there are still good reasons to believe that it helps.

Fortunately, exercise's benefits on white matter—the brain's cable system—doesn't just affect children. Exercise and training seem to boost the white matter of people, no matter their age. There is a very strong correlation between white matter in older people and how active they are. The greatest effect on white matter doesn't come from heavy-duty exercise, but rather from everyday activity and by not sitting too much. There's no need for running marathons.

You think better on your feet

It has become popular to use standing desks at the office. For most, the biggest reason for standing is probably to burn extra calories while we're working. It's true that you use up more energy while standing compared to sitting—almost twice as much—but the increased calorie expenditure is far outshined by what happens in the brain. The main benefit of standing, whether you're at school or at work, is simply that the brain functions better when you stand.

When the academic performance of seventh graders was measured using a series of cognitive tests, the kids showed clearer focus and had better working memory and executive control after they had begun using standing desks at school. The tests measured qualities that are essential for getting good grades, such as reading comprehension, remembering facts, and the ability to solve problems in several steps. The differences were significant; the test results indicated an improvement by an average of 10 percent.

Naturally, the authors weren't satisfied with only the results of these cognitive tests; they also scanned the students' brains with MRI. (My guess is that you might be noticing a pattern in these types of studies by now: first there are mental tests, followed by MRI examinations to see how the brain works.) The test results might even start to look familiar: children who had been standing before the scan just so happened to have increased activity in areas of the frontal lobe that are essential for working memory and executive control.

Scientists could see the same type of result in children who stood in class—increased activity in the frontal lobe, meaning better working memory and better focus—just like in adults and children who run, walk, or are otherwise physically active. The conclusion is simple: we think better on our feet! At school, children who stand are better at concentrating and at learning.

SMART JOCKS

Just a few years ago, not many believed that children's or adults' brains could change in such a dramatic way by engaging in physical activity. But we have learned that exercise makes us feel and tolerate stress better, it improves our memory, and we become more creative and focused. These are abilities we commonly refer to as cognitive or mental. The collective measure of all our cognitive abilities is our intelligence. If cognitive abilities are strengthened by us moving around, then exercise should increase our IQ. But is that the case? Can training make us smarter? If so, it would almost be too good to be true.

Scientists attempted to answer the question of whether exercise could increase our intelligence as early as in the 1960s, but it proved to be easier said than done. The main snag is that we don't know which is the chicken and which is the egg: if tests suggest that fit people are also highly intelligent, we don't know if it's the activity that has made them smarter, or if naturally smart people are more likely to exercise.

Data from over one million Swedish men were crucial in solving this mystery. Until a few short years ago, military service was compulsory for all eighteen-year-old Swedish males. Over the course of one trying day, a battery of tests was performed on the recruits. Among other things, endurance was gauged by having the recruit pedal to the point of failure on an exercise bike on which the resistance was continually increased. I went through the test myself, and I remember that it was incredibly hard—I could barely stand after getting off the bike. Once the biking bit was over, tests on muscle strength came next, ending with the psychological evaluation. The day of induction concluded with an IQ test.

Over the span of twenty-six years, more than 1.2 million eighteen-year-olds performed these tests. When the results were compiled recently, a very clear correlation cropped up: young men who were fit were, on average, smarter. Those who performed well on the fitness tests had a better score on their IQ test than recruits who were less fit.

Does training make us intelligent?

But was it training and fitness that made the young men smart, or did the smart recruits work out more than the others? To answer this, scientists looked at sets of identical twins. If there's one factor more than any other that can explain your IQ , it's your parent's IQ , because intelligence is, to a high degree, inherited. Identical twins have the same set of genes and have, more often than not, grown up together. When identical twins take IQ tests, their scores are typically very close within range. Among the million or so military recruits, there were 1,432 pairs of identical twins. In some cases, one twin was fit while the other was not. As identical twins, they should have had similar IQs, but they didn't. The fit twin generally scored better on the IQ test than his less fit brother. Therefore, fitness was correlated to better results on the IQ test, even among identical twins.

Collectively, everything points to the same conclusion: physical activity makes us smarter. But it's food for thought that it's only endurance—not strength—that can be associated with higher scores on the IQ test. The muscular recruits did not have better results.

The IQ test measures several types of intelligence, such as vocabulary comprehension, mathematical and logical reasoning, and the ability to see three-dimensional shapes. Good results in all these categories was associated with superior fitness. The strongest correlation was between high fitness and greater logic and vocabulary comprehension.

Today, we know that there are two areas of the brain that are especially important for logical thinking and vocabulary comprehension: the hippocampus and the frontal lobe. That the correlation was especially strong there ties in neatly with the fact that exercise's strongest effect is right on the hippocampus and frontal lobe.

Higher salary and less depression later in life

The information on the military recruits has proven to be a real gold mine for scientists in search of fascinating correlations. For example, they discovered that being fit at eighteen led to higher educational achievement and a better job with a higher salary later in life (around forty years of age). Fit young men also suffered lower rates of depression. In addition, the incidence of clinical depression seemed to be lower because

Everything points to the same conclusion: we become smarter if we're physically active!

records showed that fewer committed—or attempted to commit—suicide later in life. As if the absence of mental disorders weren't enough, other positive effects on the brain were also apparent. The physically fit eighteen-year-olds were less at risk of getting epilepsy or developing dementia later in life.

I'm not saying that all of this is because they were fit eighteen-year-olds. It's probably more the case that someone who is fit at eighteen is more likely to be a fit at thirty and forty years old.

Why is it so difficult for us to understand this?

I spend a lot of time reading scientific papers, but sometimes when I come upon this type of research, I find it hard to stay interested. It's as if I can't quite absorb it. Perhaps it just seems too good to be true that fifteen minutes of play every day can improve reading comprehension and arithmetic in children—and this without the kids even having to read or practice any of the subjects!

If you feel the same way as I do, stick around a while longer and mull over what you've just read in this chapter. Think about what it means. Let it sink in, and think of how incredible it is that children's brains not only do better academically, but function better overall if they're physically active. The brain's gray and white matter are strengthened in children who moved their bodies, just as muscles develop if you lift weights. Isn't it amazing that training can make children and adults *smarter*? That is exactly what happens! It is the best reason to encourage kids to put down their tablets and cell phones and get them to move more—because what parent doesn't want their child to become smarter and have a better-working brain?

Isn't it amazing that training seems to make children and adults smarter? That is exactly what happens! It is the best reason to encourage children to put down their tablets and cell phones, and get them to move more—because what parent doesn't want their child to become smarter and to have a better-working brain?

Have you been taken aback by the findings described in this chapter? I was, too. In fact, I was so surprised that I had to read some of the studies several times over to make sure that I had got them right.

We should ask ourselves why no one seems to know about this research. The reason could be spelled out with the letters m-o-n-e-y, as in the case of physical activity's effect on depression, which we explored in the chapter *The* real *happy pill.* If a drug, or even a dietary supplement, had shown this potency, it would have been marketed relentlessly, and we all would have heard about it. It's strange, as well as a pity, that not everyone knows that the brains of children—and of adults, for that matter—are influenced in this way by exercise. Unlike pharmaceuticals, dietary supplements, computer games, and cognitive training methods, physical activities such as playing, walking, and running are free of charge. And the body gets a "twofer" by way of a long line of positive effects that no dietary supplement in the world can match.

THE RIGHT PRESCRIPTION FOR CHILDREN AND TEENAGERS

Elevating the heart rate seems to be especially beneficial for the brain; try to get up to around 150 beats per minute.

It's the intensity that counts. Physical activity doesn't have to be about working out; play is just as beneficial. As with adults, it isn't what children *do*, it's that they do *something*.

It's best that children be active for at least thirty minutes for optimal benefits.

Shorter bouts of activity do count. When children and teenagers move around for twelve minutes, their reading comprehension and ability to focus improve. As brief as four minutes of activity at an intensity equal to jogging makes concentration easier. So, it's important to get out and play during recess, even if it's only for a few minutes!

Sporadic activity lasting ten to forty minutes at a time leads to temporary improvement in working memory, reading comprehension, and attention span.

Being physically active a few times a week for two to three months leads to permanent effects such as better arithmetic ability, increased creativity, and improved executive control (planning, initiative, concentration, and impulse control).

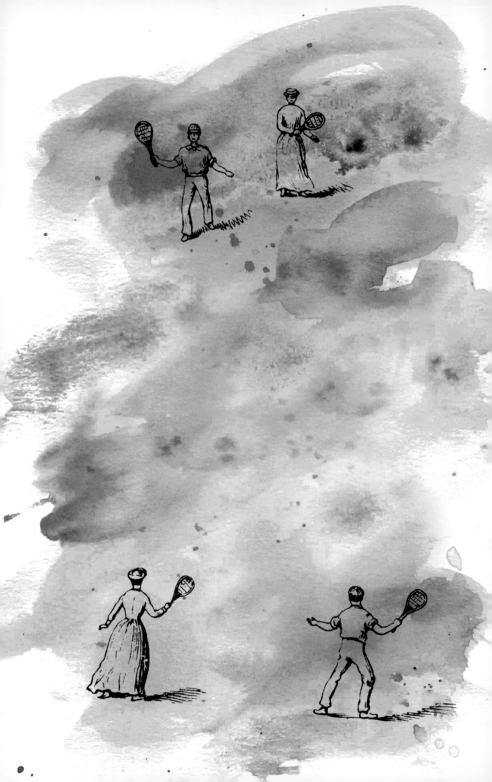

8. HEALTHY AGING OF THE BRAIN

I am physically active, walking, jogging, and running for at least four hours a day. It keeps my body and mind active.

FAUJA SINGH, 105 (who ran a marathon at the age of 100)

I'm sure we've all seen plenty of examples of how aging has big consequences on our brain's ability to function. It's not simply about our memory; at more advanced ages, we also think more slowly, and our cognitive functions such as concentration and multitasking decline. By studying how the brain works, we've begun to understand why there are differences in mental abilities between the young and the elderly.

The Stroop test consists of a word that spells out the name of a certain color—with the individual letters presented in a different color, for example, the word "blue" spelled out in red letters. You must quickly identify the color of the letters that make up the word—in this case, red—not the color indicated by the word's meaning, namely, blue. Concentration and decision making are required to suppress the impulse to choose the color specified by the word. When the brains of subjects involved in this test are examined, it shows that the anterior part of the frontal lobe, the prefrontal cortex, is activated. That is to be expected, since that part of the brain is key in decision making, focus, and impulse control.

Generally, older adults perform worse than young people on the Stroop test; they often have trouble resisting the urge to select the word color instead of the color the word is written out in, making this an effective test to call attention to the differences between the brains of the young and old.

In young brains, only some parts of the prefrontal cortex are activated, and often only on the left side. When a seventy-year-old performs the test, larger parts of the prefrontal cortex are activated, and in both sides of the brain. This probably means that the test requires more mental effort for an older person and that a larger area of the brain must be pressed into service. It's no different, really, from a young, strapping person being able to lift a chair with one arm while an older person, who might not be quite as strong, would need to use both arms.

Scientists have named this "two-brain-halves-in-use" phenomenon *HAROLD* (Hemispheric Asymmetry Reduction in Older Adults). It's interesting that one segment of seventy-year-olds that does not exhibit this tendency is made up of individuals who are physically fit. When they perform the test, only one half of their brain lights up and even smaller areas of the prefrontal cortex are involved—their brains function as if they were younger brains. Like a muscular seventy-year-old who can lift a chair with one arm, an older fit person only needs to use one side of the brain when doing the Stroop test. The test showed that they not only used less of their brain for the task; they also performed above and beyond the level of people of the same age.

THE BRAIN'S AGING PROCESS CAN BE STOPPED

The HAROLD experiment on seventy-year-olds is only one of many tests that illustrates that exercise seems to have a remarkable ability to halt the brain's aging process. As you've seen earlier in the book, the hippocampus doesn't shrink but grows in someone who is physically active. The same applies to the frontal lobe—the brain's boss. Like the hippocampus, the frontal lobe shrinks over one's life span, which adds to the impairment of our mental capacities. However, physical activity can stop the shrinking of even the frontal lobe.

In fact, the amount by which the frontal lobe contracts has been linked to how much energy (i.e., how many calories) we expend. In people who use up a lot of energy and move around, the frontal lobe seems to dwindle more slowly as they age. The thinking part of their brain—after all, the frontal lobe is where our most advanced cognitive functions are housed—is shielded from aging! By contrast, people who don't burn a lot of calories, in other words those who are very sedentary, have frontal lobes that shrink much faster. A few quick moves on the running trail is not going to make much of a difference, either; we're talking about accumulated calorie expenditure over several years here—decades, even. We can't achieve this merely by jogging sporadically around the neighborhood.

Having a wide pool of test subjects is always a good thing in medical research because it reduces the risk of getting false results. When scientists kept track of about twenty thousand women between the ages of seventy and eighty over the span of two decades, it became evident that those who exercised regularly retained their memory much longer than those who were sedentary. In addition, focus and attention were sharper in those who were active. The difference was so stark that the brains of the subjects who trained functioned as if they were three years younger. Mentally, they appeared to be, on average, three years younger than their biological age. As is so often the case when it comes to exercise's effects on the brain, we need not make Herculean efforts; a twenty-minute daily walk is enough.

THE PILOTS WHO LOST THEIR EDGE

For some individuals, having cognitive abilities that are intact isn't only essential for normal functioning; it's critical for their work. Gradually losing our ability to focus, multitask, and exhibit sound judgment as we age could mean that we are no longer able do our job. And there are few professions for which proper cognitive function is as critical as for an airplane pilot.

A team of scientists from Stanford University decided to follow 144 pilots who had to test their flying skills in a simulator on a yearly basis.

Their reactions to a series of potentially dangerous situations were observed—scenarios involved an engine failure, malfunction of the landing gear, or the presence of another plane in the wrong airspace that could send the two aircrafts on a collision course.

Points were used to grade the pilots' ability to handle these and other types of challenging situations. When they performed the test several years in a row, the results showed that flying skills gradually became impaired over time. That's no big surprise because the brain ages. However, one group of pilots' abilities declined twice as fast as the skills of the other pilots. When the scientists examined that group's genes, they discovered more incidences of a mutation of the gene for BDNF, the brain's own fertilizer. In that same group, they also noticed that the hippocampus (the memory center) had shrunk more rapidly compared to the hippocampi of the pilots who did not have that genetic mutation.

The mutation was present in one-third of the pilots, and it is estimated that about as many people in the population at large carry this gene, making the odds—ours included—of having this genetic alteration about three to one. One in three people have a gene that probably makes their brains age quicker, their hippocampi shrink faster, and their mental abilities decline more rapidly.

Is there any way to prevent this? Since you're born with a set of genes that you cannot change, if you happen to carry this gene in its mutated form, well, then it's there. However, you can strongly affect how much BDNF your brain makes—through physical activity, especially intense exercise like interval training, which provides optimal results. The scientist who conducted the study made the following statement in an interview: "There is a clear and proven way to ensure increased BDNF levels in the brain, and that is with physical activity."

We can also assert that exercise leads to improved circumstances that keep our intellectual capacities running longer in life. We can stop mental and cerebral aging. For the third of us whose genetic makeup has predestined our brain to age a little bit faster, it's imperative to get started on exercise.

Can physical activity improve pilots' flying skills? Personally, I would prefer that proper scientific evidence back things up before drawing any definitive conclusions, so at this point my answer is: let's wait and see. But there really is no reason to believe that it can't.

YOU ARE YOUR MEMORY

Of all the cognitive abilities that diminish as we age, memory stands out the most. Having a good memory is so much more than remembering where you put your keys or what was on yesterday's news. Your memory puts everything you do into perspective. Essentially, you are who you are because of your memories. Every decision you make, from the trivial— the color of your socks—to your choice of career and of where you're going to live, is tied to past experiences.

Our memory does a comparison check against past events in every situation we find ourselves in. Memory anchors us to our lives, and if our ability to remember disappears, we change as individuals. Anyone who has witnessed a person suffering from dementia will know what I'm talking about. As the ability to remember fades away, the person becomes a shadow of his or her former self. Thus, sharpening our memory entails something more fundamental than simply increasing the number of words we can recall on a memory test.

When we examine how physical activity affects memory, it's difficult to ignore the odds that we'll be diagnosed with dementia. There are more than five million Americans living with Alzheimer's Disease, a form of dementia; throughout the world, a new case is diagnosed every seven seconds. If this trend continues, there will be 150 million individuals with dementia by 2050. These figures are as grim as the illness itself.

Due to the sheer number of people affected by this disease, pharmaceutical companies have been throwing money at dementia research;

*Walking is the best medicine for
dementia!*

every year several billion dollars are earmarked for the development of
dementia drugs. Unfortunately, a cure has been elusive, and the result of
these expended billions can only be described as weak at best. As of now,
there are still no effective medications for dementia.

Walk against dementia

Scientists with far smaller budgets than pharmaceutical companies
have investigated whether there's anything that can decrease the risk for
dementia, and it just so happens that these scientists have made some
incredible discoveries. A few years ago, it was shown that a daily walk
could cut our risk of developing dementia by 40 percent. The media
didn't pay too much attention to this news, and that's a real shame
because it's a mind-boggling statistic.

A drug showing the same promise would become the world's best-
selling pharmaceutical in no time and hailed as the most groundbreaking invention since antibiotics. The Nobel Prize would be in
those scientists' pocket. We would all know the drug by name and
would probably fight tooth and nail to have it prescribed to ourselves and our loved ones to lessen our likelihood of getting dementia. As it was, the news was not about a drug but about something as
simple as going for a walk for thirty minutes, which we don't even
have to do every day—five days a week is plenty.

It wasn't only the media that missed this important discovery; a lot
of physicians did, too. Many scientists and doctors are focused on other
research, such as finding the genes responsible for Alzheimer's, the
most common type of dementia. The study of our genes is, inarguably,

thrilling, and of course there is a genetic factor to Alzheimer's, especially if you have close relatives who suffer from it. But for most of us, our genetic inheritance is less important than whether we are physically active or not. Research shows unambiguously that it is the sedentary person who needs to worry about dementia—not those who have a parent or grandparent who has the illness.

Sadly, many people for whom dementia runs in the family believe that it doesn't matter if they exercise, since they're doomed to develop the disease anyway. This is very unfortunate because it is *especially* important for them to start moving! Most of them can overcome their genetic fate, and more, with regular training.

It's truly mysterious why it has been so difficult to get this message across. It might be that genetic and pharmaceutical research is considered so very high-tech that it fires up our collective imagination, and thus makes it more media-friendly. The amazing benefit of a regular walk is pretty tame in comparison. Our initial reaction is that all that pharmaceutical money should be expected to conjure up a more cutting-edge and innovative cure than a simple walk. Well, that's not so. As it happens, walking *is* the best medicine for dementia.

A better world for the brain

How can a walk provide the best protection against dementia? It should be the brain, not the legs, that should be exercised—with crosswords, Sudoku, and different types of brain-teaser games. However, research clearly shows that a walk is *far* more important than the daily crossword, not just in protecting against dementia, but in safeguarding all cognitive abilities. Our brain does not shut off when we take a walk—far from it. Many different mental processes are engaged when we walk or run. Multiple visual impressions need to be synchronized and balanced out, while large areas of the motor cortex are busy coordinating our body's movements. Furthermore, we need to be aware of where we are and where we're going, which in and of itself presses yet more areas of the brain into service. Movement for a complicated activity, such as playing tennis, causes even more of the brain's systems to be on call. When we compare this to working on a crossword, which involves mostly the language center, we realize that the mental labor is greater when we move around than when we sit with the paper.

Besides, our brain isn't vacuum-sealed in our cranium; it is covered in a solution filled with nutrients and growth factors that is extremely fine-tuned and hugely influential on how our brain operates. To provide the brain with the best possible conditions in this bath, our blood pressure must remain stable. Likewise, blood glucose and blood fats should be in balance. The number of free radicals shouldn't be too high, and the level of inflammation in the body—there is always some level of inflammation in the body—shouldn't be excessive, either. Today, we know that all these factors are positively impacted when we are physically active, which means that the brain's environment is ideal in anyone who exercises.

The body and the brain are not two separate entities; many of the positive effects that movement has on the body—such as stable blood sugar and low levels of free radicals—strengthens the brain, as well. A strong heart will pump enough blood to provide the brain with the energy it needs. The expression "a sound mind in a sound body" isn't just a dusty cliché; it's true.

So how active do we need to be to lower our risk of developing dementia? Research has mostly defined the workload to be equal to walking or light jogging for a total of 150 minutes per week, or half an hour five times a week. Running for twenty minutes, three times a week, yields comparable results. We're not sure yet what effect weight training has on dementia, so until we know, it's better to keep doing what has proven to work: walk or run, instead of going to the gym.

It isn't only in cases of dementia that movement protects your memory. Advancing years impair memory for most of us, without having anything to do with dementia. The hippocampus shrinks, blood flow to the brain diminishes, and there's weaker contact between the different areas in the brain. But we can slow these processes down markedly if we stay active. Training slams the brakes on the brain's aging and improves our memory, whether we suffer from dementia or not.

A picture of healthy aging

The Canadian star athlete Olga Kotelko died in June 2014, at ninety-five years of age, after an incredibly successful career that included 37 world records and 750 wins. Does her name sound unfamiliar? It's no wonder: Kotelko didn't begin training at elite levels until she was seventy-seven years old. The long jump and hundred-meter sprint were two of her favorite events, and she was proclaimed the oldest long jumper in the world after her ninetieth birthday. Her field of competition narrowed in the last years of her career; in fact, she often didn't have any competitors at all. It was enough for her to turn up at the meet to be given a gold medal.

People who start training and competing in sports when they're over seventy-five years old are few and far between indeed. This is especially true for those who have never competed at elite levels before. That's why a group of scientists asked Olga if she would allow them to examine her brain by MRI. What they were looking to find out was if, and how, the brain was influenced by exercise at such an advanced age. Olga agreed to undergo the MRI, and her brain was compared to a group of her peers who had lived like most other ninety-year-olds—by resting a lot and harboring no thoughts of entering athletic competitions. The MRI showed that Olga's brain was healthier, featuring a larger hippocampus and nice-looking white matter. And it wasn't just the scans that looked good—Olga's memory was far better than those of her peers.

We can't automatically assume that Olga's brain was in better shape due to her training; it *might* already have been different right from the very beginning. However, her level of physical activity is a more plausible explanation for her brain's good health.

Olga's intense training is a perfect example of what scientists call *successful aging* of the body and brain. Olga Kotelko demonstrated that, from our brain's perspective, it is never too late to start being physically active. The brain will get stronger no matter how late in life you begin exercising. And you don't need to set your sights on breaking any world records or winning medals to obtain results.

Blue zones

There are a few regions in the world where an unusually high percentage of the population reaches the same age as Olga Kotelko—and even older—and who, like her, are untroubled by dementia. These mysterious places, which we have begun to call *blue zones*, go against the grain when compared to the rest of the world. There is a blue zone located in Sardinia, Italy, one in Okinawa, Japan, one in Costa Rica, and one in the Swedish region of Småland.

What is their secret? How can so many people reach one hundred years of age and not suffer from dementia? When scientists attempted to find the common denominator for these places, something interesting turned up. To start with, none of the blue zones are in big cities, but in small communities or on faraway islands. The people maintain strong social bonds, with several generations often living together. Very few live alone. Additionally, the people in these communities don't stuff themselves with food but consume a strict diet with fewer calories (without it being a starvation diet). Another common factor is that the populations in the blue zones are very active; their exercise tends to consist of everyday activity, not hard training.

Scientists don't know which factor (or factors) plays a part in longevity and the absence of dementia in these specific areas; it's probably a combination of several elements. What is fascinating is that people in blue zones have, on average, lower levels of education, although we know that more education is protective against dementia. That physical activity contributes to advanced age is not merely a possibility, then, but very likely. It's also interesting to note that these populations enjoy all the benefits of physical activity—long lives free of dementia—without needing to train hard. It seems that their everyday activities keep them from harm. That right there is a very good reason for taking a daily walk, for always taking the stairs, and for getting off the bus one stop or two before you reach your destination.

THE RIGHT PRESCRIPTION TO APPLY THE BRAKES ON THE BRAIN'S AGING

All activity matters! Your body takes account of every step, especially when it comes to the aging of the brain.

Walk for twenty to thirty minutes every day, at least five days a week. Or run for twenty minutes three times a week. Swimming and biking are just as good, so long as the level of exertion is the same.

Weight training is important to stay functional and mobile, but we don't know yet if it has any effect on the aging of the brain. I recommend engaging in cardiovascular training before anything else, at least until we know more about the impact of weight training.

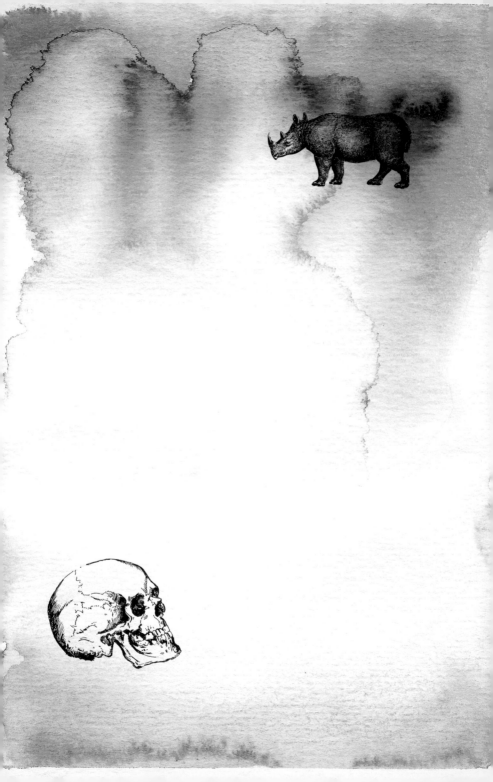

9. A STONE-AGE BRAIN IN THE DIGITAL AGE

*Nothing in biology makes sense
except in the light of evolution.*
THEODOSIUS DOBZHANSKY

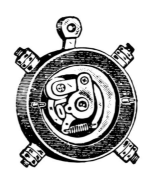

In this book, you've seen how exercise and physical activity can make you more focused, happier, and less anxious and stressed out; how it strengthens your memory; and how it makes you more creative and even seems to be able to increase your intelligence. You've discovered the mechanisms that transform your running into nothing less than a mental upgrade. Sure, it's easy to become mesmerized by the research, but personally, I believe the most thrilling aspect of it all is not *how* our brain is affected by our being physically active—but *why* it happens.

If we want to know how to make our car run smoothly, we need to understand how it is made. Same goes for the brain. If we want to make our brain function better, it's good to start by learning how it works. We don't need to become neuroscientists or psychiatrists for that. The very best way to make sense of the brain is to see how it has developed. We need to backtrack and look at the history of the brain.

We'll start from the very beginning. Lucy, whose skeleton was found in Ethiopia in the 1970s, is often considered to be our oldest known ancestor. It's believed that she lived approximately 3.2 million years ago, and that her brain volume was about 0.5 liters (just under 17 fl oz), which is a bit more than a third of today's average brain volume of 1.3 liters (just under 44 fl oz). If we fast-forward the tape by just over a million years, we'll meet *Homo erectus*, who walked upright and who was one step ahead of Lucy and her brain size. His brain's volume was just under 1 liter (1 quart), and his behavior had begun to change, too. *Homo erectus* knew how to build a fire and make tools, weapons, and clothes.

THE COGNITIVE REVOLUTION

The brain's volume started to increase at a faster pace around one million years ago. This could have been due to better nutrition, with more protein. Barely one hundred thousand years ago, our ancestors' intellectual capacity seemed to improve significantly—a phase that is commonly referred to as the *cognitive revolution*—which had great consequences. From a historical standpoint, an extremely short period saw our ancestors colonize large areas of the globe and go from being one rather inconsequential species among many others in a corner of East Africa to becoming masters of the Earth, without rival at the top of the food chain. On the way, they knocked six other human species out of the running (yes, there were at least six other different species in existence). Today, only our species, *Homo sapiens*, is still here. What made us win? We're not entirely sure, but it didn't just come from having a larger brain. The Neanderthals, for example, one of the six species we beat out, had a larger brain than ours.

One possibility is that our dominance is a result of differences in the cortex—the cerebral cortex—the outer cover of the brain. The cerebral cortex is comprised of six distinctive layers. The cerebral cortex is the center of our advanced cognitive functions. Mathematical, logical, linguistic, and creative thinking abilities can all be found in the cerebral cortex. This is the place in your brain where the magic happens. As the American astronomer Carl Sagan said, "Civilization is a product of the cerebral cortex."

A larger and more sophisticated cerebral cortex—especially the area situated behind the cranium, in the frontal lobe's anterior part (the prefrontal cortex)—translates to increased capacity and behavior flexibility.

This contributes to our big advantage for survival. We become better hunters, stronger at defending ourselves against our enemies, and, let's not to forget, more amenable to working together. All this leads to better nutrition with more protein and vitamins, which in turn gives the cerebral cortex an opportunity to evolve even further. This makes the person smarter and better still at surviving and finding food, and so on.

Today, our brain looks a bit like long, tightly packed sausages. This is to free up more room for the cerebral cortex. If the brain were as smooth and polished as a billiard ball, the overall surface of the cerebral cortex would be smaller, making us considerably more primitive.

Did a badly copied gene make us smart?

The human brain is approximately three times the size as that of a chimpanzee's, our closest relative. We split from this species six million years ago, and their brains appear to have marched in place ever since. During this time, the human brain tripled in size. Moreover, our cerebral cortex became disproportionately large compared to other animals, especially the frontal lobe and its anterior part, the prefrontal cortex.

But what was it that gave our ancestors a larger brain and an increasingly sophisticated cerebral cortex, and with it an edge over the other species? Many scientists believe the answer can be found in our genes.

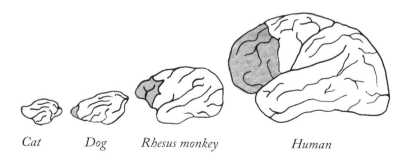

Cat   *Dog*   *Rhesus monkey*   *Human*

A STONE-AGE BRAIN IN THE DIGITAL AGE

THE BRAIN'S MOST IMPORTANT FUNCTION

In principle, only mobile living organisms possess a brain. Plants are not ambulant, so they don't have a brain. It's believed that the first brain cells were created about six hundred million years ago and that their primary task was probably to coordinate movement in primitive animals. This means that the first brain cells that emerged on Earth had movement as their most important function. At this point, the brain cells did not contribute to sophisticated brain functions like concentration, but to simpler reflexes, such as moving the organism from place to place in search of food.

The same applies to us humans. Coordination of movements has most likely been our brain's most important function, and it still is. So, if the brain's most important task is to get you to move your body, wouldn't it be odd if movement in and of itself were of no importance to the brain? The body can't move without a brain, and if the body doesn't physically move, the brain can't function as it was meant to.

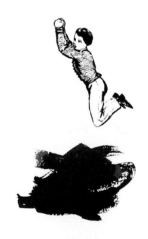

In 2015, scientists from the Max Planck Institute introduced a gene that they believe might have contributed to the fact that you are sitting here reading this, instead of scouring the savanna trying to find animals to kill.

Genes often have complicated names, and this one is called *ARHGA-PIIB*. It can be found in humans but is missing in related species like the chimpanzee. Interestingly, it looks like the gene came about purely by chance. When another gene was going to be copied in one of our ancestors, something went awry, and instead of a whole gene, only a fragment was copied. This fragment, which we today call ARHGAPIIB, had the ability to spur on the growth of the cerebral cortex. The ancestor, or ancestors, who by lucky accident was dealt the faulty genetic copy, got the slightly larger cerebral cortex, and thus the larger cognitive capacity, leading to an advantage in terms of survival. The gene was then passed down to offspring, whose cerebral cortex grew a bit more, which is how the brain has continued to develop through history.

Perhaps we have chance to thank for our intelligence. If the duplication had not been faulty and created ARHGAPIIB, we might never have made it to the moon, discovered the theory of relativity, or painted the Sistine Chapel—continuing instead to roam the savanna.

But how do we know it's just this one gene that's behind the expansion of the brain? Our genetic material contains about twenty-three thousand genes, so it could be just about any of them. Well, the answer is, of course, that it's impossible to be 100 percent sure. However, a good indication that ARHGAPIIB could very well be behind this critical evolutionary step for us humans came up after we implanted the gene in mice, which don't naturally possess ARHGAPIIB, using genetic technology.

Mice have a small cerebral cortex in relation to their body size, and the cortex has no folds; however, something happened to the mice who got the gene. They grew a bigger brain, and in several cases the cerebral cortex also showed signs of folds. In other words, their brains looked more like ours! The real, important question here is, of

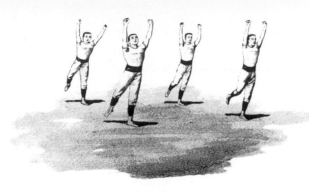

MORE MOVEMENT—BIGGER BRAIN?

Humans have a large brain compared to their body size. Its volume is approximately 1.3 to 1.4 liters (just under 44 fl oz to just over 44 fl oz), while a mammal weighing 60 kilograms (132 lbs) has an average brain volume of 0.2 liter (6.75 fl oz). This means that our brain volume is, on average, about six times as large as that of any other species. Also, an interesting correlation that scientists found when examining the brain sizes of different animals is that animals with good stamina—those that can run far—have a large brain. Like humans, rats and dogs have good stamina and, like us, they have large brains relative to their body weight.

Maybe this is because BDNF—which is created when you move—makes the brain grow and speeds up the creation of new brain cells. One possible explanation for this is that our more active ancestors were successful at finding food and surviving, and thus at propagating their genes. A lot of BDNF was generated during their physical activity, and, consequently, their brain grew. In turn, their children's brains became a bit larger, and among those offspring, those who were more physically active survived; thanks to BDNF, they also grew a somewhat larger brain, too. This is how physical activity drove the evolution and growth of the brain, which means we can thank physical activity—at least partly—for our intelligence.

course, if the mice became smarter. We don't know the answer to this yet, but we're working on it.

THE BIG SWITCH-OVER

No one is oblivious to the fact that over the last few years there's been a development where we're becoming less physical, spending more time in front of computers and smartphones. Even though this trend is as important as it is troubling, there are even more interesting connections to be found if we look further back in time. Sometime around ten thousand years ago, our ancestors turned to agriculture after having spent millions of years as hunter-gatherers. The hunter's nomadic lifestyle, with its constant, active search for food, was swapped out for a lifestyle that required staying more or less in one place. Being a farmer certainly didn't mean that you could sit around all day, but it is very likely that they were less physically active than our hunting ancestors.

The decrease in physical activity that occurred as we went from hunting to agriculture all those years ago is probably a trifle compared to what has happened over the last two hundred years, where big change has taken place in our activity habits. In just over two hundred years, we've gone from an agrarian society to an industrialized one—and today, a digitalized one—where most of us do not need to go out and actively gather food.

What was once our most important daily task over most of humanity's history has become something most of us don't have to worry about anymore, never mind being physically active in order to carry it out. Today, all our food is available at the grocery store and even online, where we can order it and have it delivered to our door to avoid having to move at all.

Half as many steps

These changes have had an enormous impact on our activity levels. Today, active people are probably far less active than the average person was two hundred years ago. So then, *how much* less active are we? It's difficult to pinpoint the amount exactly, since our ancestors did not have access to pedometers to measure how much they moved around. But by examining the activity pattern of people who still live as hunter-gatherers and comparing it to that of farmers, it's possible to make an educated guess.

The Hadza people live in north Tanzania. The tribe has about one thousand members, about half of whom live as hunter-gatherers. They have no domestic animals, they don't cultivate the earth, and they don't have permanent settlements. Instead, they subsist by hunting and building temporary shelters for the night. Their language is unique, and probably one of the oldest spoken languages on earth. Basically, the Hadza live the same way that their—and our—ancestors lived ten thousand years ago. They belong to the very last people on the planet who live as hunter-gatherers and are a rare link to our ancestors' way of life.

How active are the Hadza people? When members of the tribe were fitted with pedometers, it showed that the men walked an average of 8 to 10 kilometres (5 to 6.25 miles) a day, which is the equivalent of about 11,000 to 14,000 steps (the women walked fewer steps). That is about the same amount we believe our hunter-gatherer ancestors walked.

And what about the farmers? For reference, we can observe the Amish people in the US, an agrarian society that lives pretty much as we did two hundred years ago. The Amish have chosen to forgo all modern amenities—they don't watch television, are not connected to the internet, and don't run electricity. They move considerably more than we do. The men walk about 18,000 steps a day while the women, like the women of the Hadza tribe, take a few fewer steps. Now compare this to the 6,000 to 7,000 steps that Americans and Europeans walk daily, on average, and you'll see that the Hadza and Amish walk about twice as much as today's population in the western world. It is entirely possible that we've cut our activity pattern in half during our transition from a hunter's society to modern civilization.

In a blink of an eye

The ten thousand years that have gone by since we made the switch to an agrarian society might seem like an eternity. However, from a biological perspective, it is a very short time. Our period as farmers spans only *1 percent* of the history of humankind. The approximately two hundred years that have passed since the beginning of industrialization can also feel like a stretch, since the 1800s are undeniably long past, but from an evolutionary standpoint, it is just the blink of an eye. If we condense the history of humanity to a period of twenty-four hours, we can see that we were hunter-gatherers until 11:40 p.m. We didn't become industrialized until 11:59:40 p.m., twenty seconds before midnight. We entered the digital age (i.e., we connected to the Internet) at 11:59:59—that is, at one second before midnight!

If we consider the time it takes for other species to develop, it's obvious that evolution takes a long time. It's common that ten thousand years, and often longer, pass before anything of significance takes place, which means that today's people are generally genetically identical to those who lived one hundred, one thousand, and even ten thousand years ago.

Think about it: over a period that is basically a blip in our history, we've made gigantic changes in our lifestyle that have cut our need for physical activity in half. If we compare that to evolution's development of humanity as a species—which happens slowly, more like in terms of tens of thousands of years—you can see that our lifestyle changes have far outpaced the evolution of our bodies and brains. Evolution is lagging. Biologically, our bodies and brains are still on the savanna, and we're more hunter-gatherer than farmer. Add this to what you've read in this book so far—that your brain is strengthened by exercise; that it makes you happier, and less stressed and worried; that you become more creative and focused; that a lack of physical activity can lead you to become anxious, sad, and unfocused—and it's easy to conclude that many of today's common psychological problems stem from our lack of

If we condense the history of humanity to a period of twenty-four hours, we can see that we were hunter-gatherers until 11:40 p.m. We didn't become industrialized until 11:59:40 pm, twenty seconds before midnight. We entered the digital age (i.e., we connected to the Internet) at 11:59:59—that is, one second before midnight!

physical activity. We're walking out of step with our biological age—or, should I say, we're sitting out of step.

Why are we lazy if it's so beneficial to be active?

There is absolutely no doubt that our bodies and brains have evolved to handle activity levels far greater than we engage in today. The paradox is that we've also become lazy. If it's so good for us all-around to go outside for a walk or a run, why is it so nice to just lounge on the couch and snack on potato chips? That's because throughout most of human history, we've had to deal with an energy and calorie deficit—not an excess, like we have today. Calorie-dense meals were rare for our hunting ancestors, and it was always better to eat the food right away lest someone else tried to steal it. That's why calorie-rich foods taste so good—your brain wants you to eat all of it to fill your energy stores.

If our ancestors on the savanna came upon a tree full of sweet, calorific fruits, it wasn't particularly smart to pick one and save the rest for later, as we've been taught to do when offered a piece of chocolate from a box. For them, a better strategy was to eat it all immediately to not miss out on all those precious calories. If they waited until the next day, the fruits would probably all be gone; someone else would have taken them. That urge is still with us. For example, when faced with that box of chocolates, your brain says, "Scarf down the entire box right now, eat every little bit. Otherwise someone else will snag them! We might need

We're walking out of step with our biological age—or, should I say, we're sitting out of step.

the calories tomorrow if there's no food." That's why we feel compelled to eat the entire contents of the box.

The body's energy reserves don't depend only on how much you fill them, but also on how much energy you expend. Not using up energy unnecessarily, and being able to keep a little around the middle in reserve in case of famine, has been a survival trump card for us humans. This is an inner urge to economize our efforts and to conserve energy that can help tide us over when times are hard. So when you're lounging on the couch in front of the television, dreaming up excuses to cancel that run on the trail or the walk, it is, paradoxically, your hunter-gatherer brain that is telling you to stay put. "Sit and save energy" is the reasoning. "It'll come in handy the day there's no food, and you'll need energy."

It's obvious that this inherent urge to save calories has consequences for our weight. If you're not convinced, look at what happens in places once considered third-world countries that have experienced rapid economic growth, and that have in a few short decades given themselves over to a lifestyle full of fast food, ever-present sugar, and couch-potato TV watching. Rates of obesity have skyrocketed in these countries. It is well known that this new lifestyle causes us to gain weight, but we are not as familiar with the consequences it has on our brain.

FULL SPEED BACKWARDS!

The huge technological advancement over the last decades has given us commodities such as the Internet, smartphones, and food that can be ordered from home with the click of a mouse. Meanwhile, we're moving further and further away from the life we have evolved for. Our increased comfort makes us restless, anxious, and unhappy. Again, *why* do our mental functions suffer when we're sedentary?

Here too, the answer can be found in the past. Basically, our brain looks the same as our ancestors' ten thousand years ago. They didn't compete in marathons or work out to get in shape before swimsuit season. They were physically active simply to survive: they ran or walked in search of food, to get away from danger, and to find new places to live.

The brain is programmed to give us a kick of dopamine so we feel better if we move our body, since hunting increases our chances of survival. Moreover, those chances of survival increase if we run away from danger or discover a new area to settle down in. Since the brain hasn't changed very much over those ten thousand years, the same applies to us today. When we engage in behaviors that increased our ancestors' chances of survival, our brain rewards us with a feeling of pleasure to encourage us to repeat those behaviors.

When you come home after your run or walk, your brain interprets the activity as if you'd been out looking for food or a better place to live, for which you'll be rewarded with a feeling of well-being. You are not feeling a shot of dopamine, serotonin, and endorphins because you've read in a health magazine that it's good for you to exercise; you are getting the reward because your brain thinks you've increased your chances of survival. That's also how we're able to understand why we are "punished" by feelings of lousiness when we're sedentary. You don't catch any prey by remaining seated all day, and it doesn't lead you to find a new dwelling place, either. Being sedentary has never been good for our survival, which is why it makes many of us feel sick to this day.

In this light, it's also easy to understand why physical activity strengthens other cerebral functions. When our ancestors hunted for food, it was important that they stay focused. If you sneak up on an animal on the savanna, you need to concentrate and react to the smallest movement to boost your odds of making the kill. That's probably why you and I become more focused when we move our bodies.

Exercise also improves our memory, but how does that work? It's probably because movement has meant that we've seen new places and new environments, and it's important to be especially vigilant when we experience new things. Being sedentary and staying rooted in one spot makes the brain think that we haven't experienced or seen anything new, so there's no need to improve memory. Our brain has not evolved for us to experience new things through a cell phone or a computer; our brain does not consider sitting and staring at a screen a new experience.

The brain is still on the savanna

Your brain doesn't care that the world no longer looks like what it has evolved for. It's still very much on the savanna, and it will work a bit better if you treat it as if it were. Our exercising less is, of course, not the only change in our lifestyle and environment that affects our brain's performance and how we feel. Environmental toxins, urbanization, modern diet, and living in completely different social structures also play a role. Still, the lack of physical activity is one of the most important changes, with regards to both our physical and mental health. Our decreasing level of exercise is a problem that can be solved quite simply. While we may not be able to ditch our lives in the city and move into the woods to hunt, we can move our bodies a little more. We can take a step back to a life our brain has evolved for by becoming more active, for which our brains will offer us ample rewards.

Many of us feel that something is amiss even though we live in unprecedented material comfort. But it's not too strange that we feel this way, because our modern society has removed us far from the life we were built for. The lifestyle changes we have experienced over just a few generations have brought about incredible advantages—keep in mind how much our life span has increased. On the other hand, we tend to become depressed, anxious, stressed out, and unfocused for the simple reason that our brain has not evolved to deal with our current way of life.

You can relieve a great deal of this malaise by engaging in more physical activity. Of course, this doesn't mean that all mental problems can be solved by running on a trail or that regular tennis matches can replace all psychotropic medication. What it does mean is that most of us stand to gain a lot by exercising a little more to feel healthier and to function better mentally. If we feel low or are stressed out, maybe we should ask ourselves if there's anything in our way of life that could be altered and not automatically assume that all problems can be cured by taking a pill.

"Walking is man's best medicine"

If I were reading this book, I would be thinking by now that if exercise was truly that good for the brain, then surely everyone would be aware of it, right? It should be as widely known as the fact that smoking is bad for you and that coffee makes you perk up. I believe we've always known how good physical activity is for the brain, but over the past 150 years we've forgotten all about it. *Walking is man's best medicine.* These words are not a cliché from a health magazine; rather, they come from the mouth of Hippocrates, the father of medicine, who as far back as 2,500 years ago and without the benefit of modern medical technology understood how important moving our body was for our physical and mental health.

During the past 150 years, we've experienced staggering medical advances that have given us everything from vaccines to antibiotics, MRI scans to molecular-targeting cancer drugs. In the wake of all these amazing discoveries, everything that was obvious to us earlier seems to have fallen by the wayside. We've forgotten that the body's and the brain's most important medicine might be bodily movement. Hopefully this will change. Lately, research has caught up with Hippocrates and confirms his historic, yet wise, words. We haven't quite grasped just *how* important movement is and which mechanisms are responsible for turning a run into a mental upgrade. It's as if history were getting back at us ironically, since it is one of our most advanced medical technologies, the MRI, that has made us revisit the worth of our least sophisticated medicine—physical activity.

It's not about being a jock

Due to our current mega health hype, and because every other magazine on newsstands is a fitness magazine, tickets to events like the New York Marathon and the Swedish Vasa Cross-Country Ski Competition sell out within hours. At the same time, many people feel that they don't want or can't take part in this exercise hysteria, and I understand completely! To those, I want to say: forget about long-distance running, fitness magazines, and health hysteria, but make sure you do some type of exercise.

Being physically active isn't about being a jock or having six-pack abs; it's about providing the brain with the most advantageous conditions so it can perform at its best. Brain exercise apps have become a multibillion industry. Forget about them—they don't work. And take no notice of nutritional supplements and other "miracle methods" that are supposed to work wonders for the brain; they're ineffective, as well. Instead, spend time on what science has so clearly shown works to strengthen your brain—moving your body. And it's free. It's not important *what* you do and *where* you do it. What counts is that you do *something*. Exercise will have an immediate effect on your well-being and your mental faculties, and you will notice the biggest effects after you have worked out regularly over a longer period.

No one would be happier than I if hanging out on the couch, eating potato chips, and binge-watching TV shows were the best we could do for our brain's health. And it would be awesome if there were cognitive training methods and nutritional supplements that made me feel alert, happy, and focused all the time. Sadly, research clearly shows that this is far from reality. My brain is made for mobility. And just like yours, it will perform much better if we move our bodies!

Being physically active isn't about being a jock or having six-pack abs; it's about providing the brain with the most advantageous conditions so it can perform at its best.

10. THE RIGHT PRESCRIPTION FOR THE BRAIN

We've come to the most important part of the book, which I have left for the end. After looking at all the research on how exercise and training affect the brain, what can we define as the most beneficial activity level for the brain? How do we train to achieve maximum results? At the risk of becoming repetitive, I'll say it again: there is no exact answer to that question, but we can still draw a few conclusions.

Most important, the brain counts every step! It's better to move for thirty minutes rather than five minutes, but five minutes will count, too. Do something you enjoy!

You should walk for at least thirty minutes if you want good results.

The very best you can do for your brain is to run for forty-five minutes at least three times a week. It's also very important to raise your heart rate.

Focus on cardiovascular training. Weight training does have positive effects on the brain, but aerobic training is better. If you like working out, don't forget to include an endurance segment.

Interval training is good exercise, but less so from the brain's standpoint because you become so tired that the immediate aftereffects are less beneficial. You won't be more creative in the hours after interval training, but you will be after less strenuous training, such as running at a normal pace. That being said, interval training and other strenuous exercise is no doubt good for the brain over the long term, the reason being that intense effort strongly increases levels of BDNF.

Keep at it, keep at it, keep at it! The structural changes that come from the brain's architecture being redrawn take time. An occasional run or walk will instantly provide better blood flow to the brain, but it takes time to create new brain cells and new blood vessels, and to strengthen the connections between the different areas of the brain—months, or even longer. Those who train regularly a few times a week for six months will notice the biggest change.

208

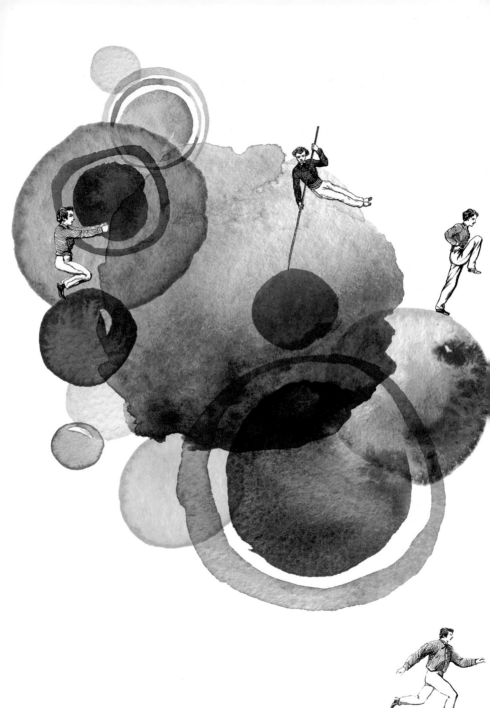

Yes, science is, in a sense, "reducing" us to the physiological processes of a not-very-attractive three-pound organ. But what an organ!

STEVEN PINKER

AFTERWORD

Inside your cranium, you have the most complex structure in the universe. An organ that is constantly active, from the day you're born until you draw your last breath. An organ that is you. Because you *are* your brain. Why have I written a book about how the brain is affected by physical activity? Well, because modern neuroscience has shown that maybe the most important thing we can do for our brain—and therefore ourselves—is to be physically active. If this is not a story worth telling, then what is, I wonder?

However, writing a science book for general readership about how the human brain is affected by bodily movement is a challenge. After all, what we're attempting to describe is an organ so enormously complex that we may never fully understand all its inner workings. Currently, neuroscience is advancing at the speed of light. Every year, about one hundred thousand scientific studies are published about the brain. That's one study every four minutes, twenty-four-seven, year-round. Our knowledge increases, literally, by the hour. Despite this, we've just begun to scratch the surface.

It took scientists forty years to map the brain activities of the small roundworm (Latin name: *Caenorhabditis elegans*), one of the animals that has been used frequently in basic brain research. That is, if it's even correct to call what it has a brain, since the tiny worm possesses about three hundred brain cells with a total of eight hundred connections between them. Compare that to a human brain's one hundred billion cells with one hundred trillion (one thousand billion) connections.

210

In other words, there's still a staggering amount we don't know about how the brain works, and not least how it is affected by exercise. In this book, I've attempted to go over the picture that neuroscience presents at this moment. No doubt future studies will reveal many new, yet unknown, mechanisms by which the brain is strengthened through physical activity. However, I'm not in the least worried that this book's main message won't still be relevant in ten or even fifty years' time. The benefits of exercise for your brain are *enormous*!

Neuroscience isn't just a way to find causes and treatments for brain diseases; it also helps us to understand ourselves. Occasionally, research has managed to confirm things that seem obvious, like how important it is for us to socialize with others, or that alcohol breaks down the brain. Sometimes the discoveries have been surprising. We don't need studies to tell us that we feel good from being physically active. However, the fact that exercise has such a big effect on our cognitive abilities (like creativity, stress tolerance, focus, and even intelligence) and that it might be one of the most important things we can do may not be quite so obvious. In fact, very few people seem to be aware of this.

This book is not about my opinions or hopes, but about science showing what *is*. At the same time, it's important for me to emphasize that this is not a scientific report, but a book on science aimed at a general audience. As such, I've had to simplify certain concepts to make the book more readable and interesting. I've included an index listing the research this book is based on, so those who want to dig deeper and get a more complete picture of how physical activity affects the brain can go to the source and find out even more. But before doing that, put down this book, and get out there and move—exercise your brain!

A MINI GLOSSARY

ACCUMBENS NUCLEUS also **NUCLEUS ACCUMBENS** A small part of the brain that is important for our reward system and for controlling our behavior. Dopamine is an important part of the nucleus accumbens, and we feel good when the levels of dopamine rise in that spot.

AMYGDALA An almond-sized area of the brain that is important for feelings of fear and emotional reactions. There are two amygdalae, one in each side of the brain. It belongs to the "reptilian brain"—the primitive parts of the brain that have remained throughout evolution. It is responsible for quickly putting the body on alert—*fight-or-flight mode!*

AXON A tendril-like offshoot from a brain cell that passes signals between the cells.

BDNF Brain-derived neurotrophic factor. A protein created by the brain that has shown to be important for many brain functions, such as creating new brain cells, as well as for our memory and general well-being.

CEREBELLUM Situated at the back of the skull, it is important for motor control and balance. The cerebellum makes up 10 percent of total brain volume.

CORTEX The cerebral cortex is the brain's outer layer and its most sophisticated part. It is also the part of the brain where major work is carried out. It consists mainly of cell bodies. The cerebral cortex is, unlike the rest of the brain, made up of six layers.

CORTISOL A stress hormone produced by the adrenal glands (situated on top of the kidneys) that increases heart rate, blood pressure, and warns and prepares us for fight or flight. In the long term, high cortisol levels will break down the brain, especially the hippocampus.

DOPAMINE A substance that controls well-being and, especially, motivation, drive, and reward. It is also important for concentration and movement.

ENDOCANNABINOIDS Endogenous substances that can produce pain relief and euphoria. They have common receptors with marijuana and THC (Tetrahydrocannbinol/cannabis).

ENDORPHINS Endogenous morphine (endogenic = originating within a cell, the body, etc.) is a group of hormones created in the brain (and the rest of the body) that can provide pain relief and euphoria.

EXECUTIVE FUNCTIONS or **COGNITIVE FUNCTIONS** A collective term for functions such as impulse control and concentration, and the ability to change and adapt behavior to current surroundings.

FRONTAL LOBE The anterior part of the brain. Logical and abstract thinking, as well as emotional control, are situated here. The frontal lobe is the most advanced part of the brain.

GABA Gamma-aminobutyric acid. A substance that calms the brain's activity.

GRAY MATTER This is mainly composed of neuronal cell bodies. The gray coloring isn't noticeable until after death. A living brain is more pink in color.

HIPPOCAMPUS Big as a thumb. There is one hippocampus in each side of the brain. Important for memory, but also for emotional control and spatial orientation. The hippocampus is the part of the brain that is probably the most affected by physical activity.

HPA-AXIS The hypothalamic-pituitary-adrenal axis is the brain's most important stress control system. It starts in the area called the *hypothalamus*, which sends a signal to the pituitary (a gland in the brain), which in turn signals the adrenal glands to produce the stress hormone cortisol.

HYPOTHALAMUS Central area in the brain important for blood pressure, heart rate, body temperature, and metabolism.

MRI Magnetic Resonance Imaging. Sophisticated medical imaging technique that displays body organs in high resolution. Functional MRI (fMRI) is used to follow different areas of the brain as they are activated. This is done by measuring blood flow to the different areas. Large blood flow indicates high activity in the area. An MRI machine is the size of a small car, and you're pushed into a tube that looks like a small tunnel. A magnetic field is created in the tunnel, and this field is so strong that the magnet that creates the field must be chilled in liquid nitrogen at a temperature of -328°F (-200°C).

NEUROGENESIS The creation of new brain cells. Earlier it was believed that new brain cells were only created in children, but now we know that new brain cells are created throughout life—even in adults.

NEURON Brain cell.

NORADRENALINE Norephinephrine. A substance in the brain that controls alertness and concentration, among other things.

ORBITOFRONTAL CORTEX Part of the cerebral cortex behind the forehead. Important for decision making and the reward system.

PET SCAN Positron emission tomography. Sophisticated medical imaging technique where radioactive substances are injected into the body. Used for research and in health care to locate tumors, among other things.

PITUITARY A pea-sized gland in the brain that regulates several of the body's important hormones like the stress hormone cortisol. The *P* in pituitary is the same *P* in the name of our body's stress control system, the HPA axis.

PREFRONTAL CORTEX Anterior part of the frontal lobe. The seat for our most sophisticated intellectual functions, like how to anticipate the future, adapt or conform to changes, put off rewards, and act toward others.

SEROTONIN A substance in the brain that is vital for our mood, especially for calm and inner strength.

SSRI Selective serotonin reuptake inhibitor. The most common pharmaceutical used in treating depressive disorders. Acts by increasing levels of the neurotransmitter serotonin in the brain but also affects noradrenalin and dopamine.

SYNAPSE The small space between two brain cells where the contact between cells happens. The cells don't touch but send out signal substances such dopamine, serotonin, and GABA to one another.

TEMPORAL LOBE The part of brain behind the temple. Important for memory, among other things.

THALAMUS Central in the brain where a lot of information passes through. Functions at times like a filter to make sure we're not overloaded with information.

THE REPTILIAN BRAIN The part of the brain that has been preserved through evolution, and that we have in common with simpler mammals. Functions like our fight-or-flight mode are there. The reptilian brain makes us react to danger (like running away) but not *anticipate* danger beforehand.

WHITE MATTER The connections between brain cells. They are situated beneath the gray matter and consist of long tendril-like axons between the brain cells. The white color is from the axons being coated in a fatty substance called *myelin* that increases the speed of signal transmission.

REFERENCES

1. Your changeable brain
Lunghi, C et al. (2015). A cycling lane for brain rewiring. *Current Biology*, DOI:10.1016/j.cub.2015.10.026.
Smith, S et al. (2015). A positive-negative mood of population covariation links brain connectivity, demographics, and behavior. *Nature Neuroscience*, 18:565–7, DOI: 10.1038/nn.4125.
Voss, M et al. (2010). Plasticity of brain networks in a randomized intervention trial of exercise training in older adults. *Frontiers in Aging Neuroscience*, DOI:10.3389/fnagi.2010.00032.

2. Run away from stress
Agudelo, L et al. (2014). Skeletal muscle PGC-1a1 modulates kynurenine metabolism and mediates resilience to stress-induced depression. *Cell*, 159(1):33–45.
American Psychological Association, 2015. Stress in America: paying with our health.
Bonhauser, M et al. (2005). Improving physical fitness and emotional well-being in adolescents of low socioeconomic status in Chile: results of a school-based controlled trial. *Health Promotion International*, DOI: 10.1093/heapro/dah603.
Colcombe, S, Erickson KI., Scalf, PE et al. (2006). Aerobic exercise training increases brain volume in aging humans. *J Gerontol A Biol Sci Med Sci*, 61:1166–70.
Dishman, R et al. (1996). Increased open field locomotor and striatal GABA binding after activity wheel running. *Physiol Behav*, 60(3):699–705.
Eriksson, K et al. (2010). Physical activity, fitness, and gray matter volume in late adulthood. *Neurology*, 75(16):1415–22, DOI:10.1212/WNL.0b013e3181f88359.
Feinstein, J et al. (2011). The human amygdala and the induction and experience of fear. *Current Biology*, DOI:http//dx.doi.org/10.1016/j.cub.2010.11.042.

Hassmen, P et al. (2000). Physical exercise and psychological well-being: a population study in Finland. *Prev Med*, 30(1):17–25.

Kim, M et al. (2009). The structural integrity of an amygdala-prefrontal lobe pathway predicts trait anxiety. *Journal of Neuroscience*, 29(37):11614–18.

Monk, S et al. (2008). Amygdala and ventrolateral prefrontal cortex activation to masked angry faces in children and adolescents with generalized anxiety disorder. *Arch Gen Psychiatry*, 65(5):568–76.

Ströhe, A et al. (2009). The acute antipanic and anxiolytic activity of aerobic exercise in patients with panic disorder and healthy control subjects. *Journal of Psychiatric Research*, 43:1013–17.

Trom, D et al. (2012). Reduced structural connectivity of a major frontolimbic pathway in generalized anxiety disorder. *Archives of General Psychiatry*, 69(9):925–34.

Zschuncke, E et al. (2015). The stress-buffering effect of acute exercise: Evidence for HPA axis negative feedback. *Psychoendocrinology*, 51:414–25, DOI:10.1016/j.psyneuen.2014.10.019.

3. Improved concentration

Beak, D et al. (2014). Effect on treadmill exercise on social interaction and tyrosine hydroxylase expression in the attention-deficit/hyperactivity disorder rats. *Journal of Exercise Rehabilitation*.

Bubl, A et al. (2015). Elevated background noise in adult attention deficit hyperactivity disorder is associated with inattention. *PLOS One*, DOI:10.1371/journal.pone.0118271.

Colcombe, S et al. (2014). Cardiovascular fitness, cortical plasticity, and aging. *PNAS*.

Eun Sang, J et al. (2014). Duration-dependence of the effect of treadmill exercise on hyperactivity in attention deficit hyperactivity disorder rats. *Journal of Exercise Rehabilitation*, 10(2):75–80.

Hillman, C et al. (2014). Effects of the FITKids randomized controlled trial on executive control and brain function. *Pediatrics*, 134:e1063–71.

Hoang, T et al. (2016). Effect of early adult patterns of physical activity and television viewing on midlife cognitive function. *JAMA Psychiatry*, 73(1):73–79, DOI: 10.1001/jamapsychiatry.2015.2468.

Hoza, B et al. (2015). A randomized trial examining the effects of aerobic physical activity on attention-deficit/hyperactivity disorder symptoms in young children. *J Abnorm Child Psychol*, 43:655–77.

Silva, A et al. (2015). Measurement of the effect of physical exercise on the concentration of individuals with ADHD. *PLOS One*, DOI:10.1371/journal.pone.0122119.

Smith, A et al. (2013). Pilot physical activity intervention reduces severity of ADHD symptoms in young children. *Journal of Attention Disorders*, 17(1):70–82.

Volkow, N et al. (2009). Evaluating dopamine reward pathway in ADHD. *JAMA*, 302(10):1084–91.

4. The real *happy pill*

Arai, Y et al. (1998). Self-reported exercise frequency and personality: a population-based study in Japan. *Percept mot skills*, 87:1371–75.

Blumenthal, J et al. (1999). Effects of exercise training on older patients with major depression. *Arch Intern Med*, 159(19):2349–56.

Dwivedi, Y et al. (2003). Altered gene expression of brain-derived neurotrophic factor and receptor tyrosine kinase B in postmortem brain of suicide subjects. *Arch Gen Psychiatry*, 60:804–15.

Fernandes, M et al. (2015). Leptin suppresses the rewarding effects of running via STAT3 signaling in dopamine neurons. *Cell Metabolism*.

Gustafsson, G et al. (2009). The acute response of plasma brain-derived neurotrophic factor as a result of exercise in major depressive disorder. *Psychiatry Res*, 169(3):244–48.

Hassmen, P et al. (2000). Physical exercise and psychological well-being: a population study in Finland. Prev Med, 30:17–25, DOI:10.1006/pmed.1999.0597.

Lang, U et al. (2004). BDNF Serum concentration in healthy volunteers are associated with depression-related personality traits. *Neuropsychopharmacology*, 29:795–98. DOI:10.1038/sj.npp.1300382.

Mammen, G et al. (2013). Physical activity and the prevention of depression: a systematic review of prospective studies. *J Prev Med*, 45(5):649–57.

Numakawa, T et al. (2014). The role of brain-derived neurotrophic factor in comorbid depression: Possible linkage with steroid hormones, cytokines, and nutrition. *Frontiers in Psychiatry*, DOI:10.3389/fpsyt.2014.00136.

Potgeiter, JR et al. (1995). Relationship between adherence to exercise and scores on extraversion and neuroticism. *Percept Mot Skills*, 81:520–22.

Rothman, S et al. (2013). Activity dependent, stress-responsive BDNF-signaling and the quest for optimal brain health and resilience throughout the lifespan. *Neuroscience*, 239:228c40.

5. Jog your memory

Chapman, S et al. (2010). Shorter term aerobic exercise improves brain, cognition, and cardiovascular fitness in aging. *Frontiers in Aging Neuroscience*, DOI:10.3389/fnagi.2013.00075.

Ericson, K et al. (2010). Exercise training increases size of hippocampus and improves memory. *PNAS*, DOI:10.1073/pnas.1015950108.

Eriksson, P et al. (1998). Neurogenesis in the adult human hippocampus. *Nature Medicine 4*, 1313–17.

Fastenrath, M et al. (2014). Dynamic modulation of amygdala-hippocampal connectivity by emotional arousal. *The Journal of Neuroscience*, 34(42):13935–47. DOI:10.1523/JNEUROSCI.0786-14.2014.

Kohman, R et al. (2011). Voluntary wheel running reverses age-induced changes in hippocampal gene expression. *PLOS One*, DOI:10.1371/journal.pone.0022654.

Leraci, A et al. (2015). Physical exercise and acute restraint stress differentially modulate hippocampal BDNF transcripts and epigenic mechanism in mice. *Hippocampus*, DOI:10.1002/hipo.22458.

O'Keefe, J et al. (1976). Place units in the hippocampus of the freely moving rat. *Experimental Neurology*, 51:78–109.

Pereira, A et al. (2007) An in vivo correlate of exercise-induced neurogenesis in the adult dentate gyrus. *PNAS*, DOI:10.1073/ pnas.0611721104.

Rhodes, J et al. (2005). Neurobiology of mice selected for high voluntary wheel-running activity. *Integr Comp Biol*, 45:438–55.

Roig, M et al. (2012). A single bout of exercise improves motor memory. *PLOS One*, DOI:10.1371/journal.pone.0044594.

Schmidt-Kassow, M et al. (2013). Physical exercise during encoding improves vocabulary learning in young female adults: A neuroendocrinological study. *PLOS One*, 8(5):e64172.

Smith, C et al. (2009). Medial temporal lobe activity during retrieval of semantic memory is related to the age of the memory. *Journal of Neuroscience*, DOI:10.1523/ JNEUROSCI.4545-08.2009.

Winter, B et al. (2007). High impact running improves learning. *Neurobiology of Learning and Memory*, DOI:10.1016/j. nlm.2006.11.003.

6. *Train yourself to be creative*

That Mozart's letter is a forgery is shown in *How to fly a horse*, a book by the American author Kevin Ashton, and in an essay by Jan Gradvall in *Dagens Industri*, May 2015.

Colzato, L et al. (2013). The impact of physical exercise on convergent and divergent thinking. *Frontiers in Neuroscience*, DOI:10.3389/fnhum.2013.00824.

Oppezzo, M et al. (2014). Give your ideas some legs: the positive effect of walking on creative thinking. *Journal of Experimental Psychology: Learning, Memory, and Cognition 2014*, 40;(4):1142–52.

Steinberg, H et al. (1997). Exercise enhances creativity independently of mood. *Br J Sports Med*, 31:240–45.

REFERENCES

7. The growing brain

Åberg, M et al. (2009). Cardiovascular fitness is associated with cognition in young adulthood. *PNAS USA*, Dec 8; 106(49):20906–11.

Burzynska, A et al. (2014). Physical activity and cardiorespiratory fitness are beneficial for white matter in low-fit older adults. *PLOS One*, DOI:10.1371/journal.pone.0107413.

Castelli, D et al. (2007). *J Sport Exerc. Psychol*, Apr; 29(2):239–52 [*sic*].

Chaddock, C et al. (2010). A neuroimaging investigation of the association between aerobic fitness, hippocampal volume, and memory performance in preadolescent children. *Brain Res*, 1358:172–83.

Chaddock-Hayman, L et al. (2014). Aerobic fitness is associated with greater white matter integrity in children. *Frontiers in Human Neuroscience*, DOI:10.3389/fnhum.2014.00584.

Davis, C et al. (2011). Exercise improves executive function and achievement and alters brain activation in overweight children: A randomized controlled trial. *Health Psychology*, vol. 30(1):91–98.

Hillman, C et al. (2009). The effect of acute treadmill walking on cognitive control and academic achievement in preadolescent children. *Neuroscience*, 159(3):1044–54.

Ma, J et al. (2015). Four minutes of in-class high-intensity interval activity improves selective attention in 9 to 11-year-olds. *Applied Physiology Nutrition and Metabolism 2014*, DOI:10.1139/apnm-2014–0309.

Martikainen, S et al. (2013). Higher levels of physical activity are associated with lower hypothalamic–pituitary–adrenocortical axis reactivity to psychosocial stress in children. *J Clin Endocrinol Metab*, 98(4):e619–27, DOI:10.1210/jc.2012-3745.

Metha, R et al. (2015). Standing up for learning: A pilot investigation on the neurocognitive benefits of stand-biased school desks. *Int. J. Environ. Res. Public Health*, 13, 0059. DOI:10.3390/ijerph13010059.

Nyberg, J et al. (2013). Cardiovascular fitness and later risk of epilepsy: a Swedish population-based cohort study. *Neurology*, 81(12):1051–7, DOI:10.1212/WNL.0b013e3182a4a4c0.

Rasberry, C et al. (2011). The association between school-based physical activity, including physical education, and academic performance: a systematic review of the literature. *Prev. Med*, DOI:10.1016/j.ypmed.2011.01.027.

Raine, L et al. (2013). The influence of childhood aerobic fitness on learning and memory. *PLOS One*, DOI:10.1371/journal.pone.0072666.

Rauner, R et al. (2013). Evidence that aerobic fitness is more salient than weight status in predicting standardized math and reading outcomes in fourth- through eighth-grade students. *The Journal of Pediatrics*, DOI:10.1016/j.jpeds.2013.01.006.

Tine, M et al. (2014). Acute aerobic exercise: an intervention for the selective visual attention and reading comprehension of low-income adolescents. *Frontiers in Psychology*, DOI:10.3389/fpsyg.2014.00575.

Van Eimeren et al. (2008). White matter microstructures underlying mathematical abilities in children. *NeuroReport*, DOI:10.1097/WNR.0b013e328307f5c1.

8. Healthy aging for the brain

Colcombe, S et al. (2006). Aerobic exercise training increases brain volume in aging humans. *J Gerontology A Biol Sci Med Sci*, 61:1166–70.

Hyodo, K et al. (2015). The association between aerobic fitness and cognitive function in older men mediated by frontal lateralization. *Neuroimage*, DOI:10.1016/j.neuroimage.2015.09.062.

Rovio, S et al. (2005). Leisure-time physical activity at midlife and the risk of dementia and Alzheimer's disease. *Lancet Neurology*.

Sanchez, M et al. (2011). BDNF polymorphism predicts the rate of decline in skilled task performance and hippocampal volume in healthy individuals. *Translational Psychiatry (2011) I*, e51, DOI:10.1038/tp.2011.47.

Tan, Q et al. (2016). Midlife and late-life cardiorespiratory fitness and brain volume changes in late adulthood: Results from the Baltimore longitudinal study of aging. *Gerontol A Bio Sci Med Sci*, DOI:10.1093/gerona/glv041.

Wueve, J et al. (2004). Physical activity, including walking, and cognitive function in older women. *JAMA*, DOI:10.1001/jama.292.12.1454.

9. A stone-age brain in the digital age

Florio, M et al. (2015). Human specific ARHGAPIIB promotes basal progenitor amplification and neocortex expansion. *Science*, DOI:10.1126/science.aaa1975.

Raichlen, D et al. (2011). Relation between exercise capacity and brain size in mammals. *PLOS One*, 6(6):e20601.

Raichlen, D et al. (2013). Linking brains and brawn: exercise and the evolution of human neurobiology. *Proc Biol Sci*, DOI:10.1098/rspb.2012.2250.

INDEX

brain plasticity, 11–17
  and stress, 55
brain programs, *see* functional
  network
brainstorming, 148, 153
brain, the
  aging of, 177–189
  damage to, 29, 43, 102
  and the memory, 128
  right side, 15
  size of, 6, 25
brake pedal for the nervous
  system, *see* GAD and hippocampus
BrdU (bromodeoxyuridine), 131,
  134, 135

C

C-14, 135–136
CAT scan, 12, 14, 90
CBT (Cognitive Behavioral
  Therapy), 54
CCK4 (Cholecystokinin
  tetrapeptid), 56
Caenorhabditis elegans, 210
calories, 169, 201–202
  expenditure, 170, 180
carbon dioxide, 45–46
cavities, *see* ventricle
cerebellum, 118
cerebral cortex, 33, 36, 70, 101,
  118, 155, 168, 193–194, 196
  motor cortex, 8
children and teenagers, the right
  prescription for, 175
chocolate, plain, 141
chronic stress, 32

Chimpanzee, 194, 196
cocaine, 100
cognitive abilities, 2, 10, 83, 98,
  142, 151, 169, 171, 180, 182,
  184, 211
cognitive functions, 5, 30–31, 74,
  142, 178, 180, 193
cognitive processing speed, 85
cognitive training, 142, 174, 206
computer game, test, 124–125,
  142, 174
concentration, 60–87
  the right prescription for, 87
  trouble with, 64
  and walking, 14
connections, 6–7, 9–11
connectivity, brain, 5, 10, 11
consciousness, 8, 70–71, 154, 155
convergent thinking, 148–149,
  154
corpus callosum (callosal
  commisure), 16
cortex, cerebral cortex, 33, 36, 70,
  101, 118, 155, 168, 193–194,
  196
cortisol, 24–30, 40, 49, 104, 128,
  166
  and grueling races, 128
Costa Rica, 187
creativity test, (Alternative uses
  test), 148
creativity, 146, 147–159
  the right prescription for, 159
crossword, 142, 184, 185
Crowe, Russell, 157
curiosity, 109
cynical, 41–42, 108, 109

tendril, *see* axon
thalamus, 71, 154–158
the right prescription
    to apply the brakes on the
      brain's aging, 189
    for children and teenagers, 175
    to feel better overall, 115
    for improved concentration, 87
    for improved memory, 143
    to increase creativity, 159
    to rid yourself of stress and
      anxiety, 57
Tyson, Mike, 47

U

UF (Uncinate Fasciculus), 35
Ullén, Fredrik, 156
ultra-runner mice, 128
ultra running, 128
Urbach-Wiethe disease, 43

V

Vasa Cross-Country Ski Compe-
    tition, 206
ventricle, 70
Vinci, Leonardo da, 70
visual attention, 165
visual cortex, primary, 7, 140
visuospatial orientation, 15, *see also*
    spatial navigation, brain GPS
vocabulary comprehension, 172

W

walk, 5, 16, 205–206, 208
    to apply the brakes on the
      brain's aging, 189
weight
    and depression, 92
    and stress, 48
weight training and memory, 140
white matter, 168–169, 173
    against dementia, 182
    and memory, 120
    to prevent anxiety, 57
Working memory, 140, 165, 170,
    175
worry, 29, 38–39, 55, *see also* stress
    and anxiety, generalized, *see*
    GAD

X

Xanax, 34

Z

Zoloft, 95–96
Zuckerberg, Mark, 147

THANK YOU!

First, an enormous THANK YOU to my brother Björn Hansen, who gave me priceless input and suggested several ideas I would never have thought of on my own. Also, a big THANK YOU to my mother Vanja Hansen, for all her encouragement and support.

Then I'd like to thank—in no specific order—the following people, who have each in their own way contributed good ideas, inspiration, and feedback during this journey: Karl Tobiesen, Simon Kyaga, Martin Lorentzon, Jonas Pettersson, Carl Johan Sundberg, Minna Tunberger, Mats Thorén, Otto Ankarcrona, Mattias Olsson, Daniel Ek, Jakob Endler, Tahir Jamil, Johannes Croner, Kristoffer Ahlbom, Gustaf Vahlne, Anders Berntsson, Erik Telander, and Lars Frick. It has been a true privilege tossing ideas back and forth with you all.

THANK YOU to graphic designer Lisa Zachrisson, who did a fantastic job boiling down my fuzzy thoughts on layout into the format of a physical book; filmmaker Alex Frey; and the editorial team at Vardagspuls.

.